From Alma-Ata to the Year 2000:
Reflections at the midpoint

To Ken Bart
Remembering our common
commitment & PHC &
HFA

Jack Bryant
Geneva 1989

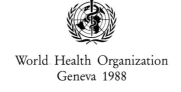

World Health Organization
Geneva 1988

ISBN 92 4 156124 6

Printed in Switzerland

88/7791—Phototypesetting—7000

Contents

Preface

The International Conference on Primary Health Care, held in Alma-Ata, USSR, in 1978, was convened in response to an international sense of despair over the widespread inequities in health and health care that afflicted all nations of the world, developed as well as developing. The conference responded with a call for radical change in both the content and design of health services, so that there would be equity in health services through primary care, thus giving rise to the highly symbolic goal of WHO — Health for All by the Year 2000.

The pronouncement from Alma-Ata had an immediate effect on the global strategies of WHO and has dominated its policies and programmes ever since. There was a somewhat delayed but nevertheless substantial impact on the health policies of the Member nations, other international organizations and nongovernmental organizations. What has been less certain is whether or not there have been improvements in health following these policy changes. What in fact has been the effect of Alma-Ata on the health of the people of the world? Have the pronouncements of Alma-Ata, the strategies of WHO, and the commitments to health for all of the Member States had a significant impact on health? Or has there been more rhetoric than reality, more ceremony than commitment?

This is far more than academic questioning. The health conditions of the poor and deprived, who exist in virtually all countries, and the costs in terms of human suffering and national underdevelopment are so extreme that the question of whether the global public health movement that began in Alma-Ata is viable or not is of the highest international significance.

The year 1988, ten years after Alma-Ata, is roughly half-way to the turn of the century. WHO, UNICEF and other interested parties decided that it was an appropriate time to review what has happened since Alma-Ata and what the prospects appear to be for the year 2000 and beyond. The Government of the Soviet Union agreed to host a return meeting, this time in Riga, capital of the Latvian Republic of the USSR. The meeting at Riga was undertaken as an assessment: "From Alma-Ata to the Year 2000 — a midpoint perspective". That meeting was held in March 1988, and its conclusions were forwarded to the World Health Assembly in May of that year.

The Forty-first World Health Assembly, to which all the Member countries of WHO were invited to send delegates, took place in May 1988 and included several relevant events:

- The document from Riga was received and considered by the Assembly.
- The Assembly celebrated the fortieth anniversary of the World Health Organization.
- A round table debate took place on the tenth anniversary of Alma-Ata, bringing together a distinguished group of people to make their observations on issues that followed from that historic meeting.
- The Technical Discussions held during the World Health Assembly were on the subject of Leadership for Health For All, a question closely related to the principles and the prospects of Alma-Ata.

The outcome of these discussions together with background materials form a substantial documentation of the views of many countries, organizations and individuals, as well as of the staff of WHO, UNICEF and other organizations within the United Nations system.

The purpose of this publication is to bring together the relevant papers, ideas, comments and questions pertaining to Alma-Ata and the problems and prospects associated with it. Efforts have been made to identify key ideas, problems and trends that might help those committed to the spirit of Alma-Ata not only to understand what has been happening but also to look ahead to the prospects for health for all through primary health care.

Many people within and outside WHO assisted the development of this publication. It found its roots in Riga, grew to maturity during the Forty-first World Health Assembly, and developed further in the weeks thereafter. The inspiration and the source of many of the most important ideas described here was, of course, Dr Halfdan Mahler, Director-General of WHO from before Alma-Ata to 1988. Important contributions were made by Dr E. Tarimo, Dr J. D. Martin, Dr D. L. Smith, and other staff of the WHO Headquarters Division of Strengthening of Health Services, including Mrs A. G. Pollinger, Mrs C. Allaman and Mrs C. Riley.

I also wish to express my appreciation to my colleagues from the Aga Khan University, Karachi, who were part of our working group at the World Health Assembly, and contributed in so many ways: Dr Mumtaz Husain, Dr Rafat Hussain, Dr Shireen Noorali, Dr Farid Midhet and Dr Asif Aslam, and our staff in Karachi, Gulshan Rajani and Darvesh Ali.

John H. Bryant, M.D.
Professor and Chairman
Department of Community
Health Sciences,
Aga Khan University,
Karachi, Pakistan

Alma-Ata: the beginning

The background to Alma-Ata

Alma-Ata is a name that has become synonymous with one of the great public health movements of history — the quest for equity in health, expressed as WHO's goal of Health For All by the Year 2000.

Not all who attended the International Conference on Primary Health Care that took place in Alma-Ata in September 1978 expected that the consequences would be so substantial or, for that matter, so controversial. But the conference was addressing an issue of great importance that had not been adequately dealt with in the past: the widespread inequities in health and health services that formed an appalling record of neglect and deprivation. It was unlikely that serious efforts to deal with such immense problems would be without reaction, negative as well as positive, from the international community of nations, organizations and individuals.

As stated by Sir John Reid, who was Chairman of the Executive Board of WHO at the time, the trail of WHO policy decisions that led to Alma-Ata began in 1974, when the World Health Assembly noted the striking disparities in health and health services between countries, and asked the Director-General to explore possibilities for more effective action. The decisions made in the Executive Board and the World Health Assembly in 1975 called for an international conference on the subject. The USSR agreed to host the conference. Then in 1977, the World Health Assembly specified that the main social target of governments and WHO in the coming decades should be the attainment by all citizens of the world by the year 2000 of a level of health that would permit them to live a socially and economically productive life. That objective was further interpreted by the Executive Board in January 1978 to mean "an acceptable level of health for all", which came to be known as health for all by the year 2000.

The Alma-Ata Conference on Primary Health Care was attended by delegations from 134 Member States and by representatives of 67 United Nations organizations, specialized agencies and nongovernmental organizations. The main documentation for the conference was the joint report by the Director-General of WHO and the Executive Director of UNICEF, entitled "Primary Health Care".

At the opening of the conference, Sir John Reid spoke as Chairman of the Executive Board and reflected on two specific dangers of any international forum. First, global pronouncements can be so general in character that they have little applicability at the level of the region or country. Alternatively, statements can be so specific that they can be applied only in a very limited number of countries or situations. The Alma-Ata Conference avoided both of those dangers and produced the Declaration of Alma-Ata, which is a truly remarkable document, every paragraph and phrase of which merits study.

The Declaration of Alma-Ata set out a challenge to WHO, the Member States and the entire world community.

Address by Dr H. Mahler, Director-General of WHO, to the International Conference on Primary Health Care, Alma-Ata, 6 September 1978

I should like to express my gratitude to the Union of Soviet Socialist Republics for having so generously agreed to host this important Conference. The Soviet Union has been a pioneer, since the first days of its Revolution more than 50 years ago, in placing health in the forefront of social goals and in linking its attainment with social justice and economic development. Its success in gradually building up the comprehensive health system of which it is justly proud was due in no small measure to the emphasis it gave to primary health care and in particular to its preventive aspects. It started with health personnel having lesser technical qualifications and expertise than their successors possess today, and it then ensured the progressive deepening of their scientific knowledge and technical skills.

Many important lessons can be learned from the evolution of primary health care and its place in the comprehensive health system in the Soviet Union, not the least of which is the harnessing of health development to social goals. Social goals vary by country — there is no universal model, as history has so dramatically illustrated — and so must the shape of health development vary by country. The health system too will be a reflection of the political and social system in which it develops and in which it is to operate. Just as there can be no universal political system, there can be no universal health system. Each country has to determine its own health system in the light of its political, social and economic realities. The motto that I have so often used, namely "don't adopt — adapt", should be our guiding principle. National self-reliance is as crucial in defining health systems as it is in defining political systems. It follows that primary health care, which in my opinion is the key to achieving an acceptable level of health throughout the world in the foreseeable future, will take a wide variety of shapes in accordance with each country's political, social and economic system. The crucial principle is that primary health care shall be widely adopted as the cornerstone to health development. Otherwise, the main social target decided upon by governments at the Thirtieth World Health Assembly in May 1977, namely "the attainment by all citizens of the world of a level of health that will permit them to lead a socially and economically productive life", will remain an empty slogan.

What can we hope to gain from this Conference? We obviously cannot cover in depth in a few days the whole range of questions relating to primary health care. What we can do is reach agreement on the main principles of primary health care and on the action that will have to be taken in countries and at an international level to ensure that it is properly understood and that it is systematically introduced or strengthened throughout the world to

become a living reality whose implementation no reactionary forces in the health world will ever be able to stop. We will discuss nationwide planning, but I must add a word of caution. I know of no country that can wait until a comprehensive integrated plan has been worked out in all its details to cover the total population. As long as there is national political determination to ensure that all citizens do enjoy the benefits of primary health care, backed by a broad national master plan to introduce and sustain it, and a sound financial basis, all entry points are valid and have to be exploited to the full wherever they are remotely feasible. Action followed by improvement within the national strategy is better than perfect planning leading to delay in action.

The successful outcome of this Conference will depend on your response to the issues at stake. I should therefore like to ask you a number of questions:

(1) Are you ready to address yourselves seriously to the existing gap between the health "haves" and the health "have nots" and to adopt concrete measures to reduce it?

(2) Are you ready to ensure the proper planning and implementation of primary health care in coordinated efforts with other relevant sectors, in order to promote health as an indispensable contribution to the improvement of the quality of life of every individual, family and community as part of overall socioeconomic development?

(3) Are you ready to make preferential allocations of health resources to the social periphery as an absolute priority?

(4) Are you ready to mobilize and enlighten individuals, families and communities in order to ensure their full identification with primary health care, their participation in its planning and management and their contribution to its application?

(5) Are you ready to introduce the reforms required to ensure the availability of relevant manpower and technology, sufficient to cover the whole country with primary health care within the next two decades at a cost you can afford?

(6) Are you ready to introduce, if necessary, radical changes in the existing health delivery system so that it properly supports primary health care as the overriding health priority?

(7) Are you ready to fight the political and technical battles required to overcome any social and economic obstacles and professional resistance to the universal introduction of primary health care?

(8) Are you ready to make unequivocal political commitments to adopt primary health care and to mobilize international solidarity to attain the objective of health for all by the year 2000?

If you emerge from this Conference inspired to respond in the affirmative to all these questions, then this Conference will have been a success. Firm in my conviction that this Conference will be a success, it only remains for me to pledge WHO's full support for the practical action that will follow.

What might be the nature of this action? I should like to suggest that all governments make an unequivocal political commitment to formulate or review their national policies and plans for primary health care within the next two years as an essential component of their development efforts. I would further suggest

5

that they ensure that national health budgets are based on these plans, in such a way as to give top priority to primary health care, and to any reshaping required in the rest of the national health system. While most of the funds will come from national sources, such programme budgets will be highly useful for mobilizing bilateral and multilateral support where it is most needed for the development of primary health care in countries, respecting fully national self-reliance.

On the basis of these national plans, and in response to their needs, WHO will be in a position to build up by no later than 1981 regional and global plans of action. These will be crucial for the strategy being developed by WHO's Executive Board for attaining an acceptable level of health for all by the year 2000. This worldwide plan of action with its national and regional variations on the central themes of the interdependence of health and development, a community-based health system and an equitable distribution of health resources leading to universal accessibility to essential health care, will be a unique manifestation of international health solidarity. But it will reach far beyond the confines of the health sector, making itself felt in many other economic and social sectors, and constituting the most important contribution of health to the establishment and maintenance of the New International Economic Order and its conversion into a truly international development order.

Finally, I should like to reassure you that my proposal for a world plan of action for primary health care as a cooperative effort of Member States is derived entirely from WHO's Constitution, which states clearly that the Organization was established for the purpose of cooperation among its Member States. This plan of action will be the epitome of technical cooperation among countries, the less affluent and more affluent working together in true partnership to define and implement a worldwide plan of action for health as part of social and economic development for all in the foreseeable future. I trust I have succeeded in conveying a message of urgency because the health situation in the world demands an urgent response. If this Conference gives rise to urgent action of the type I have outlined, it will be a decisive springboard towards better health and an improved quality of life in all countries, whatever their level of social and economic development.

I wish this Conference the success it deserves.

Declaration of Alma-Ata

The International Conference on Primary Health Care, meeting in Alma-Ata this twelfth day of September in the year Nineteen hundred and seventy-eight, expressing the need for urgent action by all governments, all health and development workers, and the world community to protect and promote the health of all the people of the world, hereby makes the following Declaration:

I.

The Conference strongly reaffirms that health, which is a state of complete physical, mental and social wellbeing, and not merely the absence of disease or infirmity, is a fundamental human right and that the attainment of the highest possible level of health is a most important worldwide social goal whose realization requires the action of many other social and economic sectors in addition to the health sector.

II.

The existing gross inequality in the health status of the people particularly between developed and developing countries as well as within countries is politically, socially and economically unacceptable and is, therefore, of common concern to all countries.

III.

Economic and social development, based on a New International Economic Order, is of basic importance to the fullest attainment of health for all and to the reduction of the gap between the health status of the developing and developed countries. The promotion and protection of the health of the people is essential to sustained economic and social development and contributes to a better quality of life and to world peace.

IV.

The people have the right and duty to participate individually and collectively in the planning and implementation of their health care.

V.

Governments have a responsibility for the health of their people which can be fulfilled only by the provision of adequate health and social measures. A main social target of governments, international organizations and the whole world community in the coming decades should be the attainment by all peoples of the world by the year 2000 of a level of health that will permit them to lead a socially and economically productive life. Primary health care is the key to attaining this target as part of development in the spirit of social justice.

VI.

Primary health care is essential health care based on practical, scientifically sound and socially acceptable methods and technology made universally accessible to individuals and families in the community through their full participation and at a cost that the community and country can afford to maintain at every stage of their development in the spirit of self-reliance and self-determination. It forms an integral part both of the country's health system, of which it is the central function and main focus, and of the overall social and economic development of the community. It is the first level of contact of individuals, the family and community with the national health system bringing health care as close as possible to where people live and work, and constitutes the first element of a continuing health care process.

VII.

Primary health care:

1. reflects and evolves from the economic conditions and sociocultural and political characteristics of the country and its communities and is based on the application of the relevant results of social, biomedical and health services research and public health experience;
2. addresses the main health problems in the community, providing promotive, preventive, curative and rehabilitative services accordingly;
3. includes at least: education concerning prevailing health problems and the methods of preventing and controlling them; promotion of food supply and proper nutrition; an adequate supply of safe water and basic sanitation; maternal and child health care, including family planning; immunization against the major infectious diseases; prevention and control of locally endemic diseases; appropriate treatment of common diseases and injuries; and provision of essential drugs;
4. involves, in addition to the health sector, all related sectors and aspects of national and community development, in particular agriculture, animal husbandry, food, industry, education, housing, public works, communications and other sectors; and demands the coordinated efforts of all those sectors;
5. requires and promotes maximum community and individual self-reliance and participation in the planning, organization, operation and control of primary health care, making fullest use of local, na-

tional and other available resources; and to this end develops through appropriate education the ability of communities to participate;

6. should be sustained by integrated, functional and mutually-supportive referral systems, leading to the progressive improvement of comprehensive health care for all, and giving priority to those most in need;

7. relies, at local and referral levels, on health workers, including physicians, nurses, midwives, auxiliaries and community workers as applicable, as well as traditional practitioners as needed, suitably trained socially and technically to work as a health team and to respond to the expressed health needs of the community.

VIII.

All governments should formulate national policies, strategies and plans of action to launch and sustain primary health care as part of a comprehensive national health system and in coordination with other sectors. To this end, it will be necessary to exercise political will, to mobilize the country's resources and to use available external resources rationally.

IX.

All countries should cooperate in a spirit of partnership and service to ensure primary health care for all people since the attainment of health by people in any one country directly concerns and benefits every other country. In this context the joint WHO/UNICEF report on primary health care constitutes a solid basis for the further development and operation of primary health care throughout the world.

X.

An acceptable level of health for all the people of the world by the year 2000 can be attained through a fuller and better use of the world's resources, a considerable part of which is now spent on armaments and military conflicts. A genuine policy of independence, peace, détente and disarmament could and should release additional resources that could well be devoted to peaceful aims and in particular to the acceleration of social and economic development of which primary health care, as an essential part, should be allotted its proper share.

* * *

The International Conference on Primary Health Care calls for urgent and effective national and international action to develop and implement primary health care throughout the world and particularly in developing countries in a spirit of technical cooperation and in keeping with a New International Economic Order. It urges governments, WHO and UNICEF, and other international organizations, as well as multilateral and bilateral agencies, non-governmental organizations, funding agencies, all health workers and the whole world community to support national and international commitment to primary health care and to channel increased technical and financial support to it, particularly in developing countries. The Conference calls on all the aforementioned to collaborate in introducing, developing and maintaining primary health care in accordance with the spirit and content of this Declaration.

Riga: Alma-Ata revisited

The background to Riga

As 1988, the tenth anniversary year after Alma-Ata, dawned, the decision was made to convene a meeting of experts from all regions of WHO as well as representatives of WHO, UNDP and nongovernmental organizations. It was to be a working meeting to bring together experts to examine the evidence and express their views on what had transpired since Alma-Ata, what the persisting problems were, and to consider what might lie ahead towards the year 2000 and beyond.

Two sets of material formed the documentation for the Riga meeting:

1. A background document[1] was prepared by Dr J.H. Bryant, entitled "From Alma-Ata to the year 2000 — reflections at the midpoint on progress and prospects". This document, prepared at the request of the Director-General, was distributed before the conference and served as a basis for discussions. The recommendations offered tentatively in the background document were modified and extended to become the definitive statement of the Riga meeting.

2. The product from Riga was entitled "Alma-Ata reaffirmed at Riga — a statement of renewed and strengthened commitment to health for all by the year 2000 and beyond".[2] It was this document, forwarded to the World Health Assembly, that served as the basis for the debate in the Assembly which led to the resolution on strengthening primary health care.

The contribution from Riga proved to be very important. It arose from the opportunity to bring together people who were widely experienced in grappling with the most serious of the world health problems, so that they could undertake a careful analysis of the impact of Alma-Ata and WHO's strategy for health for all through primary health care. The result of that analysis — "Alma-Ata reaffirmed at Riga" — helped to shape the debate and decisions of the Forty-first World Health Assembly.

---

[1] See page 14.

[2] See page 72.

From Alma-Ata to the year 2000: Reflections at the midpoint on progress and prospects[1]

... if in this world misery must exist, so be it: but let some little loophole, some glimpse of possibility at least, be left, which may serve the nobler portion of humanity to hope and struggle unceasingly for its alleviation.

Fate has allowed humanity such a pitifully meagre coverlet, that in pulling it over one part of the world, another has to be left bare.

Rabindranath Tagore, 1893 (1)

In one sense, WHO's concern for the poor is above priorities. Priorities have to do with choices. WHO has moved beyond such choices. By virtue of its own internal ethic it has permanently committed itself to serving the poor. It takes care of the world with one hand, and of the poor with the other. We have something to say about what is done with the hand that reaches to the poor.

J.H. Bryant, Karachi, January 1988

Introduction

The International Conference on Primary Health Care (PHC), sponsored by WHO and UNICEF, took place in Alma-Ata, USSR, in 1978. Decisions by the Member States at the World Health Assembly in 1977 (2), and the subsequent Declaration of Alma-Ata[2] launched the movement towards Health for All (HFA) by the Year 2000. The results have since found their place in the history of global public health movements.

What has happened since Alma-Ata? What has been the progress? The success stories? The failures? Where does HFA stand? Is the concept still alive and being worked into the fabric of health services policies and programmes? Is it still evolving in the face of new problems and insights? or has there been a fading of vision, a crumbling of resolve?

What is the agenda of unfinished effort to progress towards HFA? What are the critical obstacles? The most difficult residual tasks? The new analyses? The key targets and the priority interventions? What new resources are required? What new mechanisms? And new partnerships? What new strategies are called for?

---

[1] Taken from a background paper for the conference held in Riga, USSR, 22-25 March 1988, prepared by John H. Bryant, Professor and Chairman, Department of Community Health Sciences, Aga Khan University, Karachi, Pakistan.

[2] See page 7.

The larger question — "what have been the problems and progress in pursuing HFA since Alma-Ata?" — is immensely complex. The question has social, economic, ecological, political, biomedical and organizational aspects that apply to over 160 countries, and countless cultures and communities.

Considerable attention has already been given to these questions, most notably in WHO's global and regional evaluations of the strategy for health for all by the year 2000 (3), and in presentations by the Director-General in various fora. UNICEF's documents, particularly its annual publications on the state of the world's children, add richly to the information and policy issues involved (4, 5). The World Bank Annual Development Report is another important resource that combines detailed analysis with policy concerns (6). Sir John Reid has carefully described the sequence of events surrounding the origins and evolution of the HFA policy and programmes of WHO (7). Other observations on the HFA effort can be found elsewhere in the literature, and they will be added to extensively during this tenth anniversary year of its beginning.

Health for all — principles and imperatives

What were and are the guiding principles of HFA, and on that basis, what should be considered imperative in relation to HFA?

First, primary health care is seen as the key to achieving HFA. The original description of PHC in the Alma-Ata document of WHO is splendid and succinct (8):

> Primary health care is essential care based on practical, scientifically sound and socially acceptable methods and technology made universally accessible to individuals and families in the community through their full participation and at a cost that the community and country can afford to maintain at every stage of their development in the spirit of self-reliance and self-determination. It forms an integral part both of the country's health system, of which it is the central function and main focus, and of the overall social and economic development of the community. It is the first level of contact of individuals, the family and the community with the national health system, bringing health care as close as possible to where people live and work.

Let us point out what PHC is not:

it is not primary medical care;

it is not only first contact medical or health care;

it is not only health services for all;

and what it is and does:

it is intended to reach everybody, particularly those in greatest need;

it is intended to reach to the home and family level, and not be limited to health facilities;

15

it is intended to involve a continuing relationship with persons and families.

PHC is the key to HFA, and should include the following five concepts:

Universal coverage of the population, with care provided according to need

This is the call for *equity*. No one should be left out, no matter how poor or how remote. If all cannot be served, those most in need should have priority. Here is the *all* in health for all. Here, also, is the basis for planning services for defined populations, and for epidemiological concepts based on a population denominator that are required for, among others, determining differential needs. This principle of universal coverage may come into conflict with efforts to promote cost-effectiveness, because those most in need may be more costly to reach.

Services should be promotive, preventive, curative and rehabilitative

Services should not only be curative, but should also promote the population's understanding of health and healthy styles of life, and reach towards the root causes of disease with preventive emphasis. Treatment of illness and rehabilitation are important as well: communities rightly expect treatment services and indeed may be less interested in other services unless accompanied by curative services, and dealing with residual damage of illness through rehabilitation is an essential part of what health care can offer to support functionality and the dignity of life.

Services should be effective, culturally acceptable, affordable and manageable

Services that are not effective make a mockery of universal coverage and HFA. Ensuring effectiveness requires careful planning and management of programmes that are directly relevant to local problems. Additionally, information is required that tells PHC decision-makers what the state of the problem was at the beginning and then what has happened after intervention: without such information, the decision-maker may be blind to either success or failure in dealing with the problem. Effectiveness cannot be at the cost of cultural acceptability, indeed the two are mutually dependent. Services must be affordable in local terms, because of limited governmental resources and because the community will often have to share in the costs. And services must be susceptible to management; without effective management even well planned programmes can fall apart.

Communities should be involved in the development of services so as to promote self-reliance and reduce dependence

The community's role must be more than that of responding to services planned and designed from the outside. The community should be actively involved in the entire process of defining health problems and needs, developing solutions, and implementing and evaluating programmes. Involving the community in this way is, admittedly, often difficult and even foreign to the ways health services are usually formed. But the issue is fundamental and begs the question of whether health services are to be integral to the social development of communities, or simply another set of services provided from outside, for them to accept passively, or which they may ignore as being irrelevant to their needs and aspirations. It is this issue, the role of the community, that probably contains the greatest potential for the contribution of health to development, and at the same time is the point around which the greatest conflict is likely to arise among those with diverse points of view about how to deliver PHC.

Approaches to health should relate to other sectors of development

The causes of ill health are not limited to factors that relate directly to health, and the paths to be taken to deal with ill health must not be solely health interventions. Education for literacy, income supplementation, clean water and sanitation, improved housing, ecological sustainability, more effective marketing of products, building of roads or waterways, enhanced roles for women — these changes may have a substantial impact on health. Communities can often respond more readily to broad approaches to the problems of development than to the more fragmented sector-by-sector approach. The strength of these interactions needs to be appreciated: there are situations in which health is so inextricably tied to other aspects of development that there will be limited opportunity for advancing either health or development unless progress is made along both lines.

In reflecting on these concepts, it becomes apparent why health for all must be seen as encompassing more than health services for all, particularly when one appreciates the importance of communities developing self-reliance and of intersectoral approaches to health.

These principles and imperatives are very demanding of local, national and international systems. Beginning at the *local level*, in the community or district, much depends on the infrastructure of PHC — particularly on the personnel and how they are trained, oriented, supervised and supported — and their interaction with the community. Having facilities and staff in place is far from a guarantee of PHC that ensures equity and effectiveness. In more developed societies, services may be entirely cure-oriented and technology-intensive, with little lasting impact on health. In the Third World, the mismatch between services and needs is so common as to give rise to the often seen paradox that communities are underserved and facilities are underused.

At the *national level*, policies must be formulated that are enlightened by clear understanding of these principles and imperatives and of the PHC systems required to meet them, ideally with some field-based research capability, or at least effective feedback, that informs policy-makers about the problems that inevitably arise as planning proceeds to implementation. Policy-makers require organizational structures and capacities to extend services and support to the periphery. WHO's strong emphasis on strengthening district level health

17

services is pointed at a critical component of national HFA efforts. Budget must be there as well: policies without budgetary support become a charade. A key factor is health information systems: do people on the spot — locally or nationally — have information that tells them the extent to which their programmes have the coverage and are accomplishing what is intended? And is the information in a form appropriate for the user?

Internationally, the flow of helpful concepts, know-how and, for the poor countries, material aid is essential to quicken the pace of health development. The limited capacities of many countries to address these issues systematically, and their relative isolation from advances being made elsewhere open opportunities for creative support and communication from centres of progress to centres of need. The recent experiences of the developed countries in systematic approaches to HFA strategies and programmes are highly relevant to Third World needs. In addition, much of the most needed and relevant support and understanding can come from other developing countries which have had successful experiences in dealing with development problems (WHO refers to this as technical cooperation among developing countries—TCDC).

The demands inherent in the principles and imperatives of HFA need to be kept in view as we review the accomplishments and shortfalls of the HFA movement. Further, looking ahead we will find the need to deal with difficult problems that remain from the past, as well as entirely new problems that are already on the horizon. There will be hard choices to make, and these principles of HFA will serve as guidelines there as well.

Health for all — wistful dream or living reality?

What has been the experience with HFA? Answers are mixed, depending on where one looks, whom one asks, and what one expects.

To be sure, there have been naive hopes and false promises, but there have also been clear vision and carefully built progress. Our world is not so simple that work with highly complex problems can be summarized with "yes" or "no", and we should not reach for easy generalizations.

Let us be clear: health for all has been more than a wistful dream, captured in a slogan, supported annually from the podium of World Health Assemblies. There has been political commitment that has forced policies, budgets and programmes in support of PHC where needed. There have been medical students and faculty learning that excellence can be defined in terms of serving communities as well as in the use of sophisticated technology. These events have been spurred on by HFA. How often? In how many places? How does one quantify the diffusion of commitment and consequent action? One hears of it and reads of it in a hundred sources. One sees it in the field and knows it is real. One does it and measures it, and shows others, and they show others.

We should not forget where HFA came from. It did not spring without antecedents from WHO or UNICEF or the men and women who put the concept together a decade ago in Alma-Ata and Geneva. The underlying concepts had been taking root around the world over a number of years. It was the fact that PHC had a solid beginning in some developed countries that made it reasonable to think about commitments to improving health on a worldwide basis (9).

Further, what was now being seen as technically possible was also seen as politically and socially imperative — that the half of the world that was deprived and suffering should have hope of achieving some small part of what the other half of the world enjoyed through the benefits of affluence and modernization.

The genius of WHO and UNICEF and the Member States who led the way towards this goal of HFA was to recognize that the right moment was at hand to launch such an ambitious programme, and to identify the critical ingredients that must be involved — political commitment, ethical precepts, and technical expertise. Without political commitment, it would not be possible to set in motion the necessary policy development, budgetary allocations and shifts in priorities, all of which would require hands on levers of power. Without the ethical precepts relating to equity and need, the political commitment and technical expertise would lack a critical priority focus and the basis for social control. Without technical expertise, including science-based appropriate technology, politics and ethics would have no effective mechanisms for practical application.

But these beginnings — the stirring of what might be seen as an historic trend in health development, some emerging technology that could have large-scale applications, and insights into the social and political dynamics of the time — did not form a sure foundation for a global movement towards substantially improving the health of the world's people. Here appeared further dimensions of the genius of those who had the vision of HFA — it came in the form of directing the organizational structures and dynamics of WHO. In a decision of sheer brilliance, the headquarters of WHO turned away from the temptation of itself spelling out HFA, and threw back to the countries and regions the task of determining the purposes, content and programmes of HFA. Careful shepherding was required, but the result was a global strategy for health for all that was built from the bottom up, country by country, region by region (9). As one who was involved, at country and regional level, I remember the many sets of fingerprints that were on the various ideas and documents — the process was wide open for expressions of leadership.

What has happened since? If there is no simple "yes" or "no", it suggests there have been both successes and failures, both gains and losses. What have they been, and what do they tell us about where we are going in this quest for sensible ways to deal with the world's health?

Health for all — successes and failures, gains and losses

The range of gains and losses is very wide. One can only select a few examples that illustrate directions of impact — or lack of impact. The principles of HFA point us towards coverage with PHC as a measure of equity, and improvements in health status as a measure of effectiveness, to use those as examples. Unfortunately, there are problems in using such indicators as they may not be widely reported, and their dependability is often in question. None the less, let us see what they can tell us.

One of WHO's global indicators for monitoring progress toward HFA is availability of PHC. Most developed countries have already achieved full coverage, but even there some groups, such as poor or remote populations, have limited access. In the developing countries coverage is very inequitable, with the rural and urban poor being particularly disadvantaged. Immunization rates, which can be seen as an indicator of coverage, increased in the years 1970 to 1980 from 5% to 40% (*10*); in some countries the rates have reached ideal levels, but in a number of the least developed countries the coverage is less than 15% (*11*).

Indicators of health status tell us something about the effectiveness of programmes. The following table briefly summarizes global differences among countries in terms of under-five, infant and maternal mortality rates. The countries are grouped in order of descending under-five mortality rates, and the figures are averages for each group.

	Deaths below the age of 5 per 1000 live births	Deaths below the age of one year per 1000 live births	Maternal deaths per 100 000 live births
Very high mortality (33 countries)	211	130	450
High mortality (31 countries)	125	85	145
Medium mortality (31 countries)	108	41	90
Low mortality (34 countries)	13	10	11

Adapted from: UNICEF. *The state of the world's children, 1988*. New York, Oxford University Press, 1988.

What is dramatic here are the differences between developing and developed countries, and how wide the range is even among the developing countries. A further observation is that the differences for maternal mortality rates are even greater than for infant and under-five mortality rates. The lowest national maternal mortality rate is 2 per 100 000 live births, the highest, found in South Asia and Africa, are about 1100.[1]

But these situations have not been standing still. Changes in country status with respect to these indicators are revealing:

in 1960, there were 72 countries with under-five mortality rates of 178 or more;

in 1985, that number was halved, to 34 countries (12).

It is clear, therefore, that many countries have been making considerable and even remarkable progress in improving their health and development conditions. But others have either not improved at all, or the rates of change have been slow:

in India and Pakistan, there are more deaths of children under five than in all 46 African countries (13).

The following table shows under-five mortality rates for three periods: 1950-1955, 1980-1985 and projections for 1995-2000. Here the gains in the second half of the century are startling. But so are the residual problems — of Africa and Southern Asia, where the rates will continue to be well above 100 per 1000 live births after the year 2000.

Mortality between ages 0 and 5[a]

	1950-1955	1980-1985	1995-2000
World total	240	118	83
Developed countries	73	19	13
Developing countries	281	134	94
Africa	322	182	132
Latin America	189	88	61
East Asia	248	50	28
South-East Asia	244	111	67
Southern Asia	327	177	125
Western Asia	307	115	65

[a] The formal expression of these values is: the probability (x 1000) of a child dying between birth and the fifth birthday. This equates with the UNICEF data on under-five mortality rates.

Source: tabulations of the United Nations Population Division.

It is also important to look at indicators that go beyond health as such but relate closely to health:

the absolute number of illiterate women in developing countries is increasing, and the literacy gap between men and women is widening;

---

[1] *Maternal mortality rates: a tabulation of available information.* Unpublished WHO document FHE/86.3.

21

poverty is increasing — a billion people in the Third World are living in absolute poverty.[1]

It is apparent, then, that advances being made with HFA vary immensely from country to country and region to region. If we compare the most advanced with the least advanced countries we are comparing progress with tragedy. Some of the reasons for the differences are obvious; others are hidden in complexity. Let us first review some experiences of several groups of countries. We will then proceed to the strategic choice of giving priority attention to the poorest countries where human suffering is so immense, and the problems to be overcome are so great.

The experience of the industrialized countries

An important development in the HFA effort has been the emergence of a European regionwide strategy for HFA. In 1980, the 33 European Member States agreed to a European strategy for HFA. They set 38 HFA targets, and 65 indicators were accepted for systematic and routine monitoring by countries of national progress towards the targets (*14*). An evaluation of that strategy was carried out in 1985 (*15*).

It should be kept in mind that Europe, like North America, has been having and continues to have serious problems in paying attention to promotive and preventive aspects of health in the face of burgeoning clinical technology, rising costs and the depersonalization of medical care. The question remains open as to how much can be accomplished along the lines called for by HFA without a radical reorientation of health perspectives away from the medicalization of health that is currently dominant. This is all the more reason for the importance of this concerted effort by health leadership in Europe to develop a regionwide HFA strategy.

This process reflects how doubt and scepticism that existed prior to 1980 have given way to commitment to and confidence in the regional HFA strategy. Many Member States have made strong efforts to evaluate progress at the national level, and in a number of cases have used the opportunity to formulate national strategies in line with the regional one.

This story is all the more impressive because of a personal experience with the European Region shortly after the meeting in Alma-Ata. A number of participants at the Alma-Ata Conference were concerned that the principles of HFA would be seen as applying mainly, even exclusively, to the developing countries. With the encouragement of the Director-General and the Regional Directors, a consultation was organized in Geneva in 1979 to explore the impli-

---

[1] *Global estimates relating to the health situation and trends.* Unpublished WHO document WHO/HST/87.3, pp.33 and 39.

cations of HFA for the developed countries.[1] The organizers included Dr J.E. Asvall, the current Regional Director of WHO for Europe.

Two observations made at that consultation are worth recalling. One was that there were indeed areas in which the principles of HFA could be applied to the developed countries, and a number of such areas were identified and discussed. At one point, the representative from the Netherlands said, "If by health for all you mean that everyone has access to health services, we in the Netherlands have that; but if you mean that every one is healthy in mind and body, that is not the case. On any given day 15% to 20% of our workforce is absent from work!"

The second observation came from representatives from developing countries who thought it important to point out that the health and health services problems identified in Europe and North America — for example, hypertension and cardiovascular diseases, management and cost problems within health services — were strikingly similar to their own problems, though they would often be given different priorities.

Now that the developed countries, particularly Europe, have taken serious steps toward an HFA strategy, it is curious to look back and realize that there was once a serious question as to whether the matter even applied to those countries. This curiosity tells us how far the HFA effort has come conceptually, methodologically and politically since the time of Alma-Ata, and how far we have come in our acceptance of it. It is a tribute to WHO and its strength as an organizing force among nations that it has been able to bring about this systematic, rigorous and influential process.

Europe is not alone in the developed world in taking this direction. Canada's historic Lalonde Report (16) preceded Alma-Ata. While implementation of the concepts included in that forward-looking document moved less rapidly than had been hoped, Canada has been very progressive in the organization and financing of its health services (17).

Since 1980, the United States Public Health Service has developed health objectives for the nation (18), along lines similar to the European targets for HFA, and pursued them systematically as a national effort. Many problems are on the health agenda of the USA, including particularly dealing effectively with inequities in availability of services to people in lower socioeconomic groups, and trying to correct the effects of recent regressive policies affecting the availability and funding of services for these populations (19). On the positive side, in the United States, as in Japan and Australia, there have been striking decreases in cardiovascular and cerebrovascular mortality rates, which is in contrast to Eastern Europe, where these rates continue to rise (20).

Two final observations about the European Strategy for HFA. One is that the targets represent a deliberate attempt to change the course of European

---

[1] *Report of a consultation on health for all in the developed countries, Geneva, 1979.* Unpublished WHO document.

health development (21). This is not simply documentation of what is unfolding in health in each country, but a conscious collective effort to influence that course in favourable directions. Second is the honesty and candour with which the evaluations are undertaken. This is no whitewash, presenting merely the good side of health development. The problems, the shortfalls, and the inadequacies are described as openly as the gains. This struggle with methods and measures for improving health has important implications for the developing countries.

Those who live and work in the poorest parts of the Third World can only be impressed that this process is possible — the systematic application of the principles of HFA, and the reporting systems on which they are based (recognizing that even in Europe there are gaps and shortfalls) serve as encouraging guidelines for the developing countries.

In the Third World, embedded in the multiplicity of problems is the epidemiological transition from the diseases of infection and deficiency to the diseases of maladaptation (to use McKeown's terminology) (22). One of the truly great contributions the developed world could make to the developing world would be to provide experience-based guidance on how to avoid progressing deeply into the diseases of maladaptation, from which the industrialized nations are now trying to extricate themselves. Collaboration in this field would be intellectually exciting and of great practical significance.

Some developing countries on the move

Successes in advancing health are not limited to the developed world. There is a broad band of developing countries that have made distinct progress in dealing with their problems. Earlier we noted that in 1960 there were 72 countries with under-five mortality rates of 178 or more, while in 1985 the number was halved, to 34 countries.

Thailand is a country clearly on the move with respect to health and other aspects of development. The under-five mortality rates progressed from 195 in 1950-1955, to 61 in 1980-1985, and is projected to reach 32 by 1995-2000, according to tabulations of the United Nations Population Division. Thailand has a well organized Ministry of Health with a programme of progressively covering its population with essential health services. The extent of coverage and the effectiveness are reflected in immunization rates of 65% (third dose DPT), and a population growth rate which has been reduced to 2.2%.

Additionally, Thailand has embarked on a remarkable village-based approach to identifying and pursuing the basic minimum needs of life. Guided by an intersectoral collaboration involving the Ministries of Interior, Education, Agriculture and Health, village organizations carry out assessments of current conditions and then develop plans for desirable changes involving a broad range of community development concerns. While the process is guided from the national level, decisions and accountability are local. Here is a true community-based, intersectoral approach to the fundamental task of social development (23).

Zimbabwe stands out as an African country that is seriously addressing the problem of population growth. Strong political support plus a determined effort to monitor and manage the programme have resulted in a third of couples using contraception (24). The country has reduced its under-five mortality rate from 202 in 1950-1955 to 128 in 1980-1985, and it is projected to reach 86 in 1995-2000; immunization coverage is about 60%.

A subject that has attracted many observers of health development in the Third World is the exceptional progress made by a few countries, well beyond what might be expected from their levels of economic development. A cogent analysis of this phenomenon has been carried out by Caldwell (25). He identifies superior health achievers and poor health achievers in terms of the extent to which their levels of infant mortality are above or below that expected in relation to per capita income (he ranks countries according to per capita income and infant mortality rates (IMR); those that are 25 or more rank numbers of IMR below their per capita income rank are considered superior health achievers; those that are 25 or more ranks of IMR above their per capita income rank are poor health achievers). Each of these categories contains eleven countries. The superior health achievers have per capita incomes one-ninth of those of the poor health achievers but have achieved reductions in infant mortality rates to half the levels of the poor achievers.

He examines the characteristics of the two groups, and focuses particular attention on Costa Rica, Sri Lanka, and the State of Kerala in India, as examples of societies that have achieved major breakthroughs in health, well beyond that expected from their levels of economic development. He concludes from the experience with these three societies that unusually low mortality can be achieved if the following conditions hold:

- females receive education and have sufficient autonomy in the society that the mother can act with some independence in caring for her child and herself;

- there is a continuing political activity, especially a dominant populist or radical element, that hastens the spread throughout communities of adequate educational and health systems;

- there is ready access to health services that provide universal coverage, emphasizing maternal and child care, immunization, family planning, services provided through home visiting, and a nutritional floor of food availability.

It is clear that low child mortality will not come as an unplanned spin-off from economic growth. Caldwell emphasizes that both health services and education are required, and that there is a synergy between them. As an illustration of that thesis he presents data from studies in two Nigerian villages, where the gain in expectation of life at birth was 20% when the sole intervention was easy access to health facilities for illiterate mothers, 33% when it was education without health facilities, but 87% when it was both.

There are some differences in interpretation of various data sets and field observations between Caldwell and others, such as Mosely and Preston. Given the complexity of factors, the variations from place to place, and the changes over time, differences are not surprising. The basic point, that poor countries can achieve substantial reductions in mortality by following certain patterns of developmental activities is, of course, crucial. These kinds of observations, including the differences, are essential to the understanding necessary to make advances against what are clearly solution-resistant problems.

Poorest countries — the problem areas

It could have been predicted at Alma-Ata. Some countries have taken hold of the concepts of PHC and HFA, put forward policies, mobilized resources and implemented programmes that slowly and surely have led to improvements in the health of their populations. But other countries have not. They have not been able to establish the political base for action, pull together the necessary resources and fashion effective programmes — substantial efforts may have been there, but progress has been slow and painful; often gains against one problem have been offset by losses to another.

The reasons for these shortfalls have been many. Let us look at them in terms of politics and policy-making; problems of stagnation in national development; health services at district and local levels; health problems of the urban poor; roles of communities in health programmes; and manpower development in relation to health needs. These brief comments will introduce problems and ideas which will then be treated in greater detail below.

Politics and policy-making
At the level of politics and policy-making, policies have not been strong enough, budgetary commitments not full enough, management of health services not effective enough — one or all of these. A familiar story is that the policy commitment is made, with all good intent, but budgetary resources linked with priority for health are not there — they slip away in the give and take of cabinet-level decision-making. Health does not usually have strong leverage in national councils of power, and shifts in budgetary priorities involve shifts in power. Vision is needed at the policy-making level; the vision may be there, but not the leverage. Hard data may be required to solidify the argument, but the data are not at the policy-maker's hand, and there is no one to provide them. The opportunity passes, lost to an insistent option of another ministry.

Stagnation of development
Some countries appear to have stagnated in the development process. Scarce resources, weak infrastructures and limited management capacities weigh heavily on the development process. In the past it might have been expected that such problems could have been overcome, given time and luck. Now, new forces appear to be working, and a strong tide runs the other way.

A series of interlinked demographic, ecological, economic and political events are coalescing in some regions to produce a scary world scenario: uncontrolled population growth leads to increased pressures on land, ecological systems fail, agricultural productivity drops, per capita income falls, rural landlessness increases, internal migrants flow from rural to urban areas, political and economic instability are pervasive. This sequence and its consequences have such important implications for our concern for HFA that it is dealt with separately (see "Population growth and ecological deterioration — the demographic trap", p. 31).

Finally, there is the devastating impact of the international arms trade on health and development in the poor countries, including the reduction of development budgets to the benefit of defence expenditures.

Health services at the periphery

When policies and budgets supportive of HFA are passed along for implementation at the periphery of the health services, there may be little capacity for turning policy into effective programmes. The problems can be multiple — some deeply embedded in bureaucratic inefficiency; others caught in organizational structures that work against integration and decentralization; still others are due to lack of managerial experience, particularly in dealing with new methods and technologies of PHC. The manpower involved may not be prepared for the roles they must fill, or the support systems for them may be too weak to help them address the myriad problems at hand.

In looking broadly over the health arena, searching for weaknesses in national efforts to pursue HFA, district health systems and their management come into view as a special problem, as well as an important opportunity. Here is the peripheral organizational unit that can best serve as a channel for services to communities and as a link with more central policies and support systems. WHO is giving high priority to strengthening district health systems.

Health of the urban poor — a growing dilemma

Health problems of the urban poor seem to represent many of the worst problems of Third World underdevelopment — patterns of disease that are a mosaic of both developed and developing societies; health services that are an ineffective mixture of high technology care for those who can afford to pay, with few or no services designed to reach out to the burgeoning squatter settlements, all contained uneasily in cities whose growth is economically and ecologically unsound.

Historically without precedent, urban growth in the Third World has led to the gathering of political power within the cities, and to policies that favour urban over rural development, including concentrations of industrialization and urban subsidies that make basic goods cheaper, discourage agricultural investment, and generate accelerating rural–urban migration.

Population policies, environmental conditions, and land-ownership patterns also directly affect urbanization rates. Ineffective family planning programmes invariably result in rural populations being under pressure to migrate to cities. Where the rural environment is deteriorating as a result of deforestation, soil erosion, and desertification, cities are likely to be besieged by ecological refugees. And where land ownership is concentrated in a few hands, landlessness also drives rural people into the cities.

The cost of maintaining the cities, particularly the large urban conglomerates, is very great; bringing food and water in and getting rid of garbage and human waste are much more costly for large than small cities, and the ecological devastation of the surrounding areas is unparalleled. Indeed, the cost of maintaining the cities is a major contributor to Third World indebtedness (26).

In this milieu, the urban poor live with or die from their burdens of disease and despair. Health problems are both easier and more difficult to manage in urban areas than in rural settings: easier because of access, greater readiness for change, and more resources; more difficult because of social fragmentation, heavily contaminated environments, and political instability. But it is imperative that we learn to develop effective community-based services in these settings, because there will be no short-term reversal of the urban growth, and the needs and instabilities of these populations will increase.

The community in health development

Weaknesses at the community level involve inadequacies in the design and functions of health programmes, as well as lack of involvement of community people in deciding about and implementing health programmes.

Health programmes seldom extend beyond curative services at health centres and dispensaries to communities, and rarely reach the family level where the critical changes must take place if the health of mothers and children is to be protected. The use of community health workers (CHWs) to identify mothers and children at risk from preventable and treatable problems is usually lacking, or if present is often not backed up by front-line hospitals where there is practical understanding of the support needed. As a consequence, mothers may proceed unknowingly through pregnancy afflicted by risk factors that lead to fatal outcomes, unreported, and unseen except by sorrow-ridden families.

Communities are seldom involved in the development of health programmes beyond being expected to bring their children for immunizations, and passively to accept a thin offering of services. Governments of poor countries are often unable to provide effective services entirely free of charge, yet the resources of communities, even of poor communities, are overlooked — their capacities for cooperation, for convincing one another to change health behaviour, for supporting local health workers, for sharing in the costs of programmes, and for guiding local decisions towards the problems that are most serious and of greatest concern.

Manpower development in relation to health needs

Health personnel in the Third World are often not adequately prepared to function effectively in community-based or district-level health services. This is true of workers at all levels, but the most damaging deficiency is among doctors. Typically, the medical education of doctors, and often of nurses, is curatively-oriented and hospital-based, provided in an institution where public health and community medicine are given little attention and less respect. Such health professionals are unlikely to be useful in leadership roles that require them to relate to communities, assess needs, and plan, manage and evaluate programmes, including overseeing in-service training of other personnel. Worse, lacking such competencies but occupying the leadership role, the doctor obstructs the effective functioning of the rest of the health team.

It is probably fair to say that nursing and nursing education are not as remote from these issues as are their medical counterparts. While there are many exceptions, nursing leadership has generally been responsive to the problems and possibilities represented by HFA, and this is reflected in their literature and programmes. In the field, where there is a public health and PHC orientation, nursing is often the mainstay of the service.

There are serious deficiencies in the material and psychological support that health workers at the periphery receive. They often have the justifiable sense of working in isolation — that there are no serious efforts to provide them with the basic amenities required to live and raise a family in a relatively remote setting; that there is limited concern for ensuring provision of the elementary materials and back-up required for them to be effective; and most damaging of all, that they and the work they are doing are not respected, even within their own health field. The resulting demoralization is widespread and deeply damaging.[1]

Looking ahead—priority choices

Viewing the full canvas of WHO and its goal of HFA for the world's people, it is quite clear that its Constitution, organizational structures and participatory relationships with the Member States make it both possible and mandatory for the Organization to relate to all the major problems of the world — but not with equal concern and attention. WHO is, after all, the organizational embodiment of commitment to equity — universal coverage, and care according to need. True, all countries need, use and contribute to the work of WHO, but most are not deeply dependent on the Organization; some are. For some, the dependence on external assistance is extreme, linked to survival itself.

This is not a new story for WHO. It is accustomed to swinging priorities towards need, urgency, and suffering. Here, we propose that WHO focus priority attention on the least developed countries, and we will suggest aspects of their problems that call for special attention, with special urgency, and with new directions of programmatic thinking.

The remainder of these comments will follow that priority trail of concern for the least developed countries. We will try to delineate some of their most serious problems, then we will discuss several avenues for intervention.

---

[1] *Report of the interregional meeting on strengthening district health systems based on primary health care, Harare, Zimbabwe, August 1987.* Unpublished WHO document WHO/SHS/DHS/87.13.

The least developed countries: critical problems

In considering the problems of the poorest countries, we will focus our attention on two approaches to defining their problems: first, using indicators of mortality and morbidity; and second, a concept of development-gone-wrong, the demographic trap.

High rates of morbidity and mortality

No single measure of health status can capture the nature and extent of health problems; problems are too complex to be measured so simply, and there are so often exceptions to the applicability of any one indicator. None the less, mortality rates of mothers and children signal the daily tragedies of life and at the same time reflect many other aspects of underdevelopment.

Maternal and under-five deaths are distributed between developed and developing countries as follows (27):

	Maternal deaths	Under-five deaths
Asia	310 000	8 090 000
Africa	150 000	4 200 000
Latin America	34 000	1 010 000
Developed countries	6 000	300 000
World	500 000	13 600 000

These data show that only a very small proportion of maternal and under-five deaths occur in the developed world, around 1 or 2%.

Looking now at the countries, we can aggregate the poor countries into two groups:

33 countries with combined populations of 477 million with an under-five mortality rate over 170 per 1000 live births;

31 countries with combined populations of 1520 million with an under-five mortality rate between 95 and 170 per 1000 live births.

These 64 countries have 40% of the world's population but more than 80% of infant and child deaths and more than 90% of maternal deaths. It is these 64 countries that we suggest be given priority attention. What can we say about the mortality data of these countries?

Deaths of infants and small children are due mostly to diarrhoeal disease, acute respiratory infections and immunizable diseases, generally complicated by and contributing to malnutrition. These conditions are most prevalent where there is poverty, illiteracy (particularly of women), large families, contaminated environments and inadequate health services. These factors often interact, reinforcing one another, in vicious turns of malnutrition and infection, heightening the likelihood of infant and childhood death (28, 29). The problems are exacerbated in times of famine and social or political instability. Generally speaking, these problems can be prevented and/or cured through low-cost, community-based health activities, many of them provided in the home, supported by an appropriate range of health facility-based services.

Maternal deaths are due largely to infection, haemorrhage, toxaemia, obstructed labour, unsafe abortion and other complications of delivery.[1] While the immediate or direct causes of maternal mortality are listed above, many aspects of a woman's life in the Third World add to the risks: poverty, illiteracy, frequent pregnancies, undernutrition, anaemia, heavy workloads. The point is that it is the conditions of life that so often place these women at risk of death. These various causes of death can generally be prevented or treated through low-cost, community-based health services, together with referral arrangements to a district facility where complications can be managed.

Population growth and ecological deterioration— the demographic trap

Considerable attention has been given to the recession of the mid-1980s, which has been so damaging to the economies of Third World countries, particularly in Africa. A penetrating analysis of an extension of this problem has been developed by Lester Brown of the World Watch Institute (30); it warrants consideration in some detail because of the profound implications for our concern for HFA.

Brown begins with Notestein's theory of demographic transition, which was built largely on the European experience:

first stage—both birth and death rates are high and the population grows slowly if at all;

second stage—living and health conditions improve and death rates fall, but birth rates remain high and the population grows rapidly;

third stage—economic and social gains combine to reduce birth rates, and, as in the first stage, birth rates and death rates are in equilibrium, but at a much lower level.

This has been a highly useful conceptualization, but a gap has appeared in the analysis — what happens when countries get trapped in the second stage, unable to achieve the economic and social gains necessary to reduce births? What happens when second-stage population growth rates of 3% per year begin to overwhelm ecological life-support systems?

Three areas of development reversal occur: population growth exceeding the carrying capacity of ecosystems; declining agricultural productivity and

---

[1] *Preventing the tragedy of maternal deaths: a report on the International Safe Motherhood Conference, Nairobi, February 1987.* Unpublished World Bank/WHO/UNFPA document.

incomes; and rural landlessness. These combine to trap nations in the second stage of the demographic transition. Let us look at several contributing factors.

We now have *a demographically divided world*: half of the world where population growth is slow and living conditions are improving, and half where population growth is rapid and living conditions are deteriorating. The slow growth countries are increasing at 0.8% per year and adding 19 million people per year to their populations. Rapid growth countries are growing at 2.5% per year and adding 65 million people per year.

Countries with rapid and sustained population growth are in danger of exceeding, or are already exceeding, the carrying capacity of their ecosystems, the result of which can be a collapse of the biological capacity of the land to support the population. In countries where population growth remains high, a three-stage ecological transition emerges that is almost the reverse of the demographic transition since it is the end-stage that is disastrous:

> *first stage*—expanding human demands are well within the sustainable yield of the biological support system;
>
> *second stage*—human demands are in excess of the sustainable yield, but are still expanding as the biological resource itself is being consumed;
>
> *third stage*—human consumption is forcibly reduced as the biological system collapses.

Once populations expand to the point where their demands begin to exceed the sustainable yield of local forests, grasslands, croplands or water systems, they begin to consume the resource base itself. Forests and grasslands disappear, soils erode, land productivity declines, water tables fall, wells go dry. This in turn reduces food production and incomes, triggering a downward spiral.

Since 1973, when oil prices increased, the growth of the global economy has slowed markedly, a decline that is extreme when expressed in per capita terms for the poorer countries with high population growth rates. During the 1970s, Africa became the first region since the great depression to experience a decade-long decline in per capita income, and all indications are that the situation will worsen through the 1980s. Latin America is likely to join Africa in that trend, and the subcontinent of Asia is not immune to the same possibilities.

An important part of this global economic slowdown was the loss of momentum in agriculture. Per capita grain production is now declining in some 40 developing countries. The combination of diminishing agricultural productivity, the requirement for importation of foods, and external borrowing with heavy costs of debt servicing presses countries into situations from which it is extremely difficult to emerge.

Growing rural landlessness is still another emerging problem affecting Africa, Asia and Latin America. The largest landless populations are in South Asia, where 40% of all rural households are landless, and indications are that the problem will worsen. The landless have far higher levels of malnutrition, lower levels of education, and lower life expectancies than others in society. This landless class, often outside the mainstream of development and bereft of hope, is also a potential source of social and political unrest. The relationship between population growth and social conflict is not well understood, but will call insistently for better understanding in the years ahead.

In 1986, a murderous riot broke out in a crowded squatter settlement of Karachi. More than 250 people were killed, thousands were injured and hundreds of homes were gutted. This blood-spattered event, which largely victimized innocent people, was thought to arise from drug and gun trafficking, but the stage was set by crowding from rural-urban migration, poverty, and despair that quickly gave way to anger.

For many Third World countries, the demographic trap is becoming the grim alternative to completing the demographic transition. The long-term alternative becomes a return to the equilibrium of the first stage — with high birth rates and death rates. Such a regression is already evident in Africa, where famine has raised death rates twofold since 1970. In short, countries may already have lost the chance to escape from the demographic trap.

The problem statement

We have laid out two ways of defining the problems of the poorest countries — through maternal and under-five mortality rates, and by putting forward observations about the demographic trap.

These definitions of problems are deliberately chosen to throw up two quite different signals to those concerned about HFA strategies. One—maternal and under-five mortality rates — are reasonably clear and unequivocal descriptors of what must be considered unacceptable levels of health of the most vulnerable of the world's population, and WHO and its Member States must use their expertise to find ways to deal with these problems. The problems result from poverty, ignorance, contaminated environments, ineffective and inefficient health services, inappropriately trained and utilized health personnel, and scarcity of leadership. This is not to say that dealing with these issues will be easy, but the directions to take are not obscure.

The other — the demographic trap, an example of development-gone-wrong — has an entirely different import. Taken as presented, a number of developing countries are at risk of proceeding into development disasters. The nature of the disasters and the factors that contribute to them are complex, even confusing, largely because they cross boundaries that most of us, at least in the health sector, are unaccustomed to seeing in juxtaposition: population growth, ecological carrying capacity, agricultural productivity, landlessness, falling per capita incomes, and social and political instability. And health is there too, embedded, as one of the ingredients of disaster. Many of these are new issues; and while there has been a great deal of research on individual components, the integration of this knowledge, particularly of the overall impact of newly emerging effects, still lies ahead.

WHO speaks of intersectoral relationships and health — and here it is, with startling meanings. Unlike the problem of high under-five and maternal mortality, however, the ways into this problem are much less clear. This is unfamiliar territory. The causal factors seem less susceptible to control. New research agendas are just now being formed. Addressing these problems would call for entirely new strategies, partnerships, resources, and on an entirely different scale. And the costs of failure are higher.

Of course, one could say the analysis of the demographic trap is false, that the problem does not and will not exist. But there is another reason for putting forward the demographic trap as a problem to be considered in the context of future strategies for HFA. Consider it to be a paradigm of development-gone-wrong, where the current rules for dealing with health problems no longer fully apply, the disciplines so carefully built by the health sector are not adequate to define the problems, and the problems have different kinds of complexity. Here, we see evidence of health standing on too narrow a base of both concept and practice. Different coalitions of disciplines, agencies, countries and resources will be needed. And different time scales are involved.

A final word about the future and its predictability. We should not allow ourselves the luxury of thinking in terms of surprise-free futures. We must be ready for surprises: pleased if they are pleasant ones — say, science's gift of an effective AIDS vaccine; and prepared if they are destructive. If the demographic trap does not turn out to be as bad as it might be, there will be others — war, famine, continuing and worsening poverty. Let us be ready with a new generation of organizational structures, interdisciplinary and cross-sectoral partnerships, conceptual road maps, and field-based research sites.

These, then, represent two problem areas, against which we can test our thinking, our strategies for moving effectively on the problems we can see, and for preparing for the problems that we cannot yet see, but which will probably supervene.

Fresh strategies for a new era

In dealing with the poorest countries and most difficult problems, we — the concerned people of the world — are in a very different position than we were at Alma-Ata in 1978:

- We know a great deal about how to build health programmes around the concepts of PHC.
- We have gained important advances in applicable technology.
- We have important experiences in diagnosing our own failures.
- We know where the most resistant problems lie — by country, social class, ecological setting.
- We have some successful models to guide us.
- We have leaders in both developing and developed countries who have demonstrated success in dealing with tough problems.

At the same time, we know that much more must be done than has been done if there is to be an ameliorating impact on the most tragedy-ridden countries and communities. New approaches are needed, and they are needed with a sense of urgency.

- We must move on a scale and at a pace beyond those of the past.
- We need to seek new ways of analysing the problems, and new ways of describing the problems to facilitate broader appreciation of their nature.
- We need to seek new mechanisms, new partners, new resources for dealing with the problems.
- We need to develop more effective ways of convincing people about the needs, the problems, and the possible solutions.

But answers will not come easily. We are now dealing with a hard core of solution-resistant problems. There will be few magic bullets, quick fixes, technological miracles. Answers will come only through careful, sustained long-term efforts, not through parachuted aid packages. Most of the efforts must be directed at building the capacities of the countries involved: their systems, their manpower, their infrastructures, their leadership — not only at national level but also at community and intermediate levels.

We will now examine five subject areas. Each can be considered a critical avenue for addressing the broad health problems of the poorest countries, but we will give special consideration to maternal and under-five mortality, and to the paradigm represented by the population growth-ecosystem deterioration, the demographic trap. The five areas are:

- strengthening political and social interventions;
- strengthening the organization and management of health systems, particularly in districts;
- supporting community-based and home-based health activities;
- facilitating applications of science and technology to PHC; and
- developing leadership for HFA.

Strengthening political and social interventions

Just as current flows of resources, both nationally and internationally, will not be adequate to address the difficult health problems, so current mechanisms for directing resources toward those problems will fall short of what is required. There is an imperative need for social imagination that will identify and construct new mechanisms and new partnerships for these purposes.

The continuing spread of HFA

There is no doubt that WHO has been highly successful in eliciting formal statements from all Member States in support of the meaning and intent of HFA. Indeed, looking region by region, an amazing number of countries have gone well beyond endorsement of HFA through WHO to actually shaping their own national strategies around the precepts of HFA:

- in Bangladesh national health policies are built around the precepts of HFA, and a National HFA Council is being set up to conduct periodic reviews of HFA strategies (*31*);

- in Mongolia, HFA strategies have been fully incorporated into the national socioeconomic plan (*31*);

- in Chile, a Council of Ministers responsible for social areas has been organized to adopt HFA as a policy at the highest level of government, and to coordinate the solution of problems relating to health and the quality of life (*32*);

- Finland, Sweden and Yugoslavia have developed clear national strategies based on HFA (*33*);

- Spain has passed a new general health law based on the principles of HFA (*33*);

- Mexico has taken the remarkable step of amending its Constitution to establish health care as a right of citizenship (*32, 34*).

As an entirely different kind of sign of international diffusion of the idea of HFA, statements concerning the principles of HFA, such as equity, universal coverage and the importance of PHC, have become pervasive in nongovernmental as well as governmental circles. In many countries, developing as well as developed, statements based on HFA appear in policy documents, local newspapers, magazines, titles of papers at symposia, speeches by politicians, and public relations releases by policy offices. Yes, at the level of political commitment and popular statement, HFA has taken root.

The uncertain commitment to HFA

The troublesome questions have to do with the extent and effectiveness of both commitment and implementation. We can rightly worry that the concept of HFA may simply solicit responses in support of HFA that are, in reality, lip-service without deep commitment to the values and actions that are called for. Let us look at these problems of limited commitment, first at the international, and then at national levels.

What is the international climate for support of HFA and development? Unfortunately, that climate is often, and in many places, ice-cold. Perspectives that centre on materialism rather than equity; on narrow views of economic development rather than longer-term needs for social development; lack of understanding of or confidence in the processes of development, or even outright contempt for the people of developing countries, find their ways into development policies. Some of these tendencies are aggravated during times of recession, as in the downturn in the world economy of the early 1980s.

Developing countries suffered from the world recession of 1980—83 to an almost unprecedented extent, including worsening trade and the building up of an intolerable debt burden. The resulting imbalances led to a need for major economic adjustment in many countries. Unfortunately the form of the adjustment policies adopted frequently contributed to worsening conditions among vulnerable groups. Income per head fell in 17 out of 23 countries in Latin

America, and in 24 out of 32 countries in Africa. There has also been widespread deterioration in the health status of vulnerable populations, including mothers and children (35).

The major mechanisms by which adjustment policies tend to worsen conditions for the most vulnerable include: reducing employment for low-income households; increasing prices of basic commodities, especially food; and reducing government expenditures on basic services, such as health, education and sanitation.

While there is increasing recognition of the negative effects of such adjustment policies, this period is reflective of how health and other aspects of development fall victim to shifts in economic policy that focus almost exclusively on economic as opposed to broader aspects of social development.

Turning to the national level, one place for probing the depth of commitment is in terms of budgetary allocations to health, as well as agency commitment to programme implementation aimed at equity and coverage with PHC. If one tries to follow the trail from policy about HFA to implementation of PHC programmes, the tracks often fade rather quickly. The health budget is often tiny — 1-5% of total national expenditure; and even the published budget may be a political figure and not reflect funds actually available for expenditure (36).

While the health budget may be small, the part committed to PHC and related efforts is often disproportionately even smaller. Efforts to move resources from hospitals and speciality services to PHC for the urban and rural poor often run into powerful opposition. Of course, even when the resources are there, earmarked for PHC, they may not be well used — a dismal story in itself.

Political commitment is an uncertain commodity. Well-meaning political figures may not have freedom of action within their party or administration. Political constellations of power may be transient, and what was solid accomplishment today may evaporate tomorrow.

Searching for new resources, new partners, new mechanisms to support HFA

A vital issue is how the interests, commitments and resources of a broader constituency of support for the poorest people and poorest nations can be mobilized. It is clear that current approaches — plans, programmes, resources, time-frames, scales of action — will not break through the intractability of the most difficult problems. Indeed, it is likely that a continuation of current approaches will have diminishing effects, because the resources are losing value, and the problems are exacerbating. There is a need to move with different partners, different sources of support, to use different mechanisms to bring all pressures to bear on the problems.

It needs to be seen very clearly that the resources required for development support have not been coming from the international transfer of funds from the developed to the developing countries. In Africa, the net transfer of funds shrank from US$ 8.6 billion a year over the 1977—78 biennium to minus US$ 5.4 billion in 1984—85. In Latin America, the shift was even greater, from US$ 4.9 billion a year in 1977—78 to minus US$ 39 billion in 1984—85 (35).

While mechanisms are being sought among donors and recipients to ameliorate this extraordinary problem of debt burden, the outlook is surely one of great fiscal constraint for the years ahead.

What are some of the other directions that can be explored in order to address the serious and solution-resistant problems of the poorest countries? To begin, it is important to appreciate the substantial contributions made to health and social well-being by the nongovernmental sector: voluntary organizations, nongovernmental organizations, universities, religious organizations, industry, foundations and numberless individuals. A difficult but important task would be to quantify the numbers and resources they represent. An effort to analyse resources available for development from both governmental and nongovernmental sources has been carried out by WHO's unit of Health Resources Mobilization.[1]

An interesting development is the emergence of very large numbers of organizations and institutions that are indigenous to the developing countries (voluntary agencies, religious organizations, foundations). Literally thousands of socially oriented indigenous groups exist, many of them waiting for indications of useful directions in which to apply their energies and resources.

The nongovernmental organizations (NGOs) have extremely varied memberships, purposes, resources, modes of function and levels of effectiveness. The potential of these organizations is very great, both for direct programmatic action and also for political leverage. In view of the limited effectiveness of many governmental programmes, the NGOs have a special role to play in constructive criticism of weak or faulty governmental programmes as well as in the development of prototypes that they or governments might use and expand.

Just as current flows of resources, both nationally and internationally, will not be adequate to address the difficult problems, so current mechanisms for directing resources towards those problems will fall short of what is required. There is a need for social imagination that will identify and construct new mechanisms and new partnerships for these purposes.

Social and political activism are not new, to be sure, but new uses of these fundamental societal forces will be extremely valuable at local, national and international levels, through which concerned people and organizations can bring their views and the power of their positions to bear on ineffective, misguided and exploitative agencies and officials.

---

[1] *Donor profiles: a guide to official development assistance agencies.* Unpublished WHO document COR/HRM/86.2.

Women's organizations have a special part to take in support of health and development programmes aimed at the care of women, children and families. The UN Conference on Women and Development held in Nairobi in 1985 resulted in an outpouring of interest, enthusiasm and ideas that far exceeded expectations. The organizational infrastructure that evolved in relation to that event is still intact, with the possibility of reactivation around critical issues of women and development.

Regional groupings of countries have potential for assisting the poorest countries, particularly when resource-rich countries are involved. The Association of South East Asian Nations (ASEAN) is an example, with Japan as one of the participants. The ASEAN Centre for Research and Training in PHC of Mahidol University, Thailand, is a product of Japanese support in the context of South-East Asia.

At an international political level, why should it not be possible for some of the largest nations to join in a collaborative effort to assist some of the poorest countries? The USSR and the USA have had long-standing agreements for cooperation in biomedical science, with exchanges of scientific delegations and collaborative research. This cooperation has weathered a number of diplomatic conflicts between the two nations, clearly because each wanted to keep this relatively non-political interaction alive. Thus far, the exchanges have not extended directly to interaction with the Third World. In view of the recent disarmament treaties, and with prospects for further steps in disarmament, it would be an extraordinary step for the two nations to agree to explore the possibilities of joint assistance in development to some of the poorest countries. Here would be a symbol of immense importance if the two nations not only agreed to such joint action but also indicated that the resources involved would be taken from savings derived from reduced expenditures on arms.

An example of a different kind of mechanism is that developed by The Pew Foundation (USA), WHO and the World Bank, which addresses one aspect of health policy-making in developing countries. They have put together a programme directed at supporting policy-makers who require research-based information for policy formulation. This International Health Policy Research Program helps countries to establish mechanisms for policy dialogue and policy-related research efforts. Making the best use of resources for PHC is an expected focal point of the programme. Here, then, is an example of a new mechanism, new resources, and a new coalition of partners who are assisting in the furtherance of PHC and HFA (37).

Those who do not appear to hear, see or care

While calling to mind the people, organizations and institutions who are striving for new mechanisms to deal with these difficult and often tragic problems of development, it also needs to be said that there are many organizations and institutions that do not appear to hear or see or care about the needs of the deprived and destitute populations. Universities, including or perhaps even especially medical schools, have been surprisingly aloof from and sceptical of the HFA effort. Health professionals of various kinds, many large hospitals, politicians and numberless private citizens appear to be so deeply engaged in their own affairs as not to be able to raise their heads and eyes to see the needs of the poor.

One feels the need to shout out to those who exploit the poor: the weapons merchants; the drug runners; the politicians who pay lip-service to social need in order to ensure their election and power base; those who profit commercially from products that are threats to health, whether infant formulae, tobacco or pharmaceutical mixtures designed for profit and not for the patient's well-being; and doctors who organize their practices to maximize profit without corresponding concern for patient welfare.

Defence budgets, often presented as justifiable in terms of internal and external threats to national security, escalate to 10, 20, even 30 times the health budget. Large defence budgets have highly destructive effects on the social and economic conditions even of the rich countries (38). When a poor country spends 3 to 30 times more on defence than on health, it means that not enough is left to cover even the barest requirements of life for the most vulnerable part of the population.

If there is a clearly visible enemy of society, with strong evidence to show the irrationalities of its purported intent, it is the war machines of both developing and developed worlds.

Strengthening the organization and management of health systems, particularly in districts

While acceptance of PHC is fairly general at policy levels in the poorest countries, implementation of effective programmes that achieve widespread coverage is hardly ever seen. The problem is only partly due to scarcity of resources. There are serious weaknesses in planning, management, financing and evaluation capacities, and in the training of personnel and providing effective support for them in field settings.

More attention needs to be given to the development of the health services infrastructure — facilities, manpower, management, information systems, logistics — which is needed to support a variety of PHC programmes. Here is a critical issue in health services development — given an effective infrastructure, PHC programmes can be added or deleted according to local need (39).

Related to infrastructure development there have been conflicts and competition between selective (or vertical) and integrated approaches to PHC, but that problem may now be receding (see discussion below).

A further weakness of health services has been the lack of supportive interaction between the district and higher levels of health services on the one hand, and between district and community level activities on the other. At national or regional levels, strongly centralized decision-making discourages initiative at the district level. At district level, the focus of interest in facilities and doctor-based services, together with limited orientation toward community involvement, result in little support to community-level activities.

In pointing out these shortfalls, one needs to be careful about unrealistic expectations. In most of the poorer countries, the leadership capacity is of a high order of commitment and competence, but the possibilities for implementation of effective PHC programmes at field level are very limited. One must deal with very simple, very practical systems that can reach large numbers of people with readily implementable interventions. Immunization is the best example of what needs to be done, where the technology and management are known and well communicated, yet the shortfalls are many. None the less, the Expanded Programme on Immunization (EPI) is taking root, and other programmes can follow, benefiting from the infrastructure and programme management required for EPI.

Despite these problems, there is immense potential for health services based on PHC to progress toward the goals of HFA. Much of the basic technology has been worked out. Many dozens of examples or prototypes of such services are established and working. Some countries have applied them on a widespread basis: Botswana, Costa Rica, Indonesia and Thailand are among the many examples. The challenge is to work these systems into place in the poorest countries.

The needs for effective health services based on PHC are so great, and the potential for improvement so extensive that a discussion of strategies could be difficult to contain. Here, we will focus on four areas that represent both problems and opportunities.

Measuring effectiveness and locating accountability

A fundamental and pervasive problem in health services is an inability and even disinterest in determining morbidity and mortality rates, or other indicators that would define the baseline state of problems and provide a basis for evaluating programme effectiveness. Infant and young child mortality rates are rarely known at a local level, and national rates are aggregated figures with little local meaning. The practical consequence is that programme managers, or simply health teams, do not know how many lives are being lost and how many are being saved.

The same can be said for other measures — of coverage with services, and prevalence and incidence of problems such as malnutrition, low birth weight, rates of contraceptive use, complications of pregnancy. These, linked with process and outcome measures, are strong guides in the management of health services, and their omissions are symptomatic of serious and widespread deficiencies of perspective and method in PHC systems.

It might be said, of course, that these measures require methods that are too complex for the usual health services. They need not be. One of the challenges is to develop simplified systems for community surveys that can be carried out by ordinary health teams and community people, to use simple indicators that can serve as proxies for more complex measures, and to use such indicators to guide the development of health services. The analysis of data can be done with pencil and paper and hand calculator.

In Pakistan, there is an urban PHC programme in which community health workers (CHWs) visit families on a monthly basis and report on immunization status, nutritional status (weight for age and weight change), maternal status, and births and deaths. This simple, low-cost system allows the health team to monitor coverage and effectiveness of PHC programmes, and to know when they are succeeding or failing. The information system showed that there was success in the immunization programme but children were dying due to malnutrition and infectious complications. Knowledge of this failure led to changes initiated by the CHWs, who worked out methods of convincing mothers to feed their children differently — the prevalence of serious malnutrition is now decreasing. This PHC system, including the surveillance component, is affordable and manageable in the Pakistani context.

Related to the lack of data to indicate coverage or effectiveness is the lack of placement of accountability for success or failure of programmes. Who is responsible? Who is counting? Who are counted? The community might well ask, are we worth counting? The combination of lack of evaluative data, and the lack of placement of accountability results in systems that are blind to their effectiveness, or lack of it, and powerless to correct drift or failure.

Here is the heart of HFA's challenge — equity. Without a system design that can achieve coverage, without simple indicators to tell of success or failure, without effective management (including a capacity for self-correction), without involving the community in these processes, equity becomes a charade.

Health manpower:
under-prepared, under-supported, demoralized
At the centre of the weaknesses of health services based on PHC is manpower. So often, in so many places, local health professional leadership which could guide and shape such health services is missing. The deficiency is deep and widespread — with professionals inadequately trained and not motivated to work where the needs are.

There are two sides to the manpower equation. One is that recruitment and training are too often separated entirely from utilization — a reason for WHO's long time emphasis on health services and manpower development (HSMD) as a unified concept. The story of training of health personnel that is both inadequate and irrelevant to the tasks that must be carried out is so often told as to require no repeating here (see Developing leadership for health for all, page 55).

Less well appreciated is the severe demoralization of health personnel that is apparent in so many field settings, particularly in the more peripheral locations. The neglect and unresponsiveness of the health services with respect to these people is consistent, widespread and destructive of their potential for effectiveness. Several factors can be emphasized:

- lack of well managed and disciplined health services that provide opportunities for accomplishment, that are both personally gratifying and professionally rewarding;
- lack of material incentives to compensate for work in difficult settings; personnel being so underpaid as to make outside and possibly unsanctioned work mandatory;
- lack of opportunities for professional advancement, with little prospect for intellectual or position betterment;
- lack of professional recognition and respect, often even within their own professional field;
- lack of arrangements congenial to family life, including education of children;
- lack of dynamic interaction with communities that would add social and spiritual rewards to the professional work;
- lack of social and professional solidarity that can come from effective functioning as a team.

In aggregate, these factors often lead to a sense of uselessness and lack of motivation, and, when such despondency occurs, loss of dependability and integrity is not far behind. This is not a problem of system design, nor is it necessarily inherent in PHC systems. Rather, it has to do with management practices and personnel support systems that are insensitive to human needs.

This bleak picture is not universal, but it is widespread enough to warrant careful attention. **It makes no sense to preach social sensitivity and self-reliance for communities, when the same sensitivity and support are not directed towards the health personnel who must effect those developments in the communities.**

Selective v. comprehensive PHC

There has been an uneasy and at times divisive debate over two approaches to providing health services in the poor countries, namely selective or vertical programmes versus integrated or comprehensive PHC systems (40). Currently, proponents seem to be shifting positions, generally towards a middle ground, and the matter might be left at that, but the issues are so important that they are worth reviewing briefly.

The selective side of the debate began with the observation that the PHC approach is too idealistic to be implemented by most governments. Instead, it is more realistic to target scarce resources to control specific diseases that account for the highest mortality and morbidity, particularly where there are available low-cost technologies for prevention and treatment.

The other side of the debate, put forward in favour of integrated or comprehensive PHC, involves establishing a community-based infrastructure for PHC, and addressing the health problems through appropriate PHC programmes in the context of overall development, with the communities actively involved in the planning and implementation.

One of the reasons for heightened concern about these issues is that the selective approach fits the technological and political orientation of some donor agencies who look for concrete objectives and measurable outcomes, achieved in a relatively short period of time; in embracing these characteristics of selective programmes, they might ride roughshod over fundamental principles of community-based PHC. Those concerned with this approach should be wary of the following:

- pursuing individual disease problems with a specialized infrastructure that either would not add to or would be duplicative of the more general PHC structure;
- focusing on health exclusive of other aspects of development;
- by-passing community involvement in deciding which programmes should be selected and in their implementation;
- focusing on short-term processes when some of the important community development processes are necessarily long-term.

The position we take here is that health must be seen as part of overall development, that the community must be involved in that development process, indeed the community is the instrument and object of development, and that the strengthening of community capacities to cope with development problems has important consequences for the quality of the lives that are saved through PHC. The development of a PHC infrastructure is critical: developed side by side with communities, it provides a mechanism for involving the community, for responding to community needs and concerns, for adding or subtracting PHC programmes according to decisions made within the community, and for introducing appropriate technologies into a local PHC setting. Obviously, these concerns do not diminish the possibilities of using technologically strong methods for analysis and control of diseases (39).

District health systems based on PHC

The recently established emphasis of WHO on strengthening district health systems (DHS) is well placed to have a critical impact on the HFA effort in the priority countries.

A DHS may be considered to be the local operational framework required for the implementation of PHC. It is an integral part of the national health system, including a population living within a clearly delineated administrative or geographical area, whether urban or rural. It includes all institutions and individuals providing health care in the district, whether governmental, social security, nongovernmental, private or traditional. The principal features of a DHS based on PHC can be listed:

- it is based on equity in relation to need;
- it provides accessibility and coverage to entire populations;
- it emphasizes health promotion and disease prevention;
- it addresses intersectoral determinants of health as well as health services;

- it seeks to involve and empower communities and individuals to assume greater responsibility for their own health;
- it uses an integrated approach for more efficient use of scarce resources;
- it gives attention to incentives and motivation of teams of health workers.

The district can play a pivotal role in matching local needs and priorities with national policy guidelines and resource allocations. Playing this role effectively requires adequate decentralization to the district of both responsibility and resources. Both community involvement and intersectoral action can take place at various levels within the DHS. The district has the potential to improve the integration of various programmes within the health services, such as the resolution of the problem of selective programmes v. integrated PHC. The district can also promote more coordinated efforts of various governmental, private, voluntary and community groups.

Focusing on district health systems in relation to PHC provides an essential mechanism for probing the factors that have a bearing on difficult problem areas such as maternal and young child mortality and the interactions of population growth and ecological deterioration. Study of the latter problem, of course, will call for special choices of geographic and ecological conditions, but there will still be overlapping interests and methods. In particular, the nexus of family life and environmental circumstances — how couples make decisions about the spacing of children and the size of families, and how mothers care for their children — is central to both sets of problems.

One of the most difficult linkages to establish among the various levels of health services is between hospitals and PHC systems, and it is especially difficult where it is most important — between the front-line or district hospital and community-based PHC. Without close interaction, the community-based services are on their own without direct support and uncertain about referral, and the hospital functions in traditional isolation, not knowing and having no way of knowing the relevance and effectiveness of its services in relation to the needs of the surrounding population. This linkage is a key piece that is missing in the development of effective services (41), and the district health system is an ideal place to pursue it.

The district offers opportunities for working out how planned programmes, including those that are community-based, can address these critical problems. WHO's approach of engaging interested countries and NGOs in a network of collaborating districts offers an extremely interesting mechanism for international cooperation in this field. A key requirement of such work is to be locally specific, because the causes and solutions must be locally based, culturally and ecologically; at the same time workers must be able to compare and carry lessons from one place to another.

It can be noted as well, how these arrangements may involve new organizational mechanisms for addressing problems, new partners in collaboration, and a larger scale of action both locally and internationally.

Supporting community-based
and home-based health activities

While universal literacy is an essential long-term goal, informal education has its place as well. In societies where education comes with difficulty and marriage is early, talented and able women may still have to sign their names with a thumb print. They need to be identified and given opportunities for self-improvement and to contribute to the development and quality of life in their communities.

There is a paradox about the roles of communities in PHC. The importance of community involvement in health services is widely expounded, but actual involvement is much less apparent. When one is on the front line trying to implement PHC programmes for poor populations in the Third World, the reasons for the paradox become clearer; it is much more easily said than done. But it is essential. Without community involvement, the services provide only packaged programmes that community people can accept and use, or reject and not use, as they decide.

Involvement of communities in PHC is not a social nicety, it is a technical necessity. PHC programmes cannot achieve coverage and effectiveness without the full involvement of communities. The key advances in the health of communities depend on their decisions — whether or not to be immunized, to feed children differently, to use family planning, to use oral rehydration therapy properly, to seek and use clean water, to control environmental contamination, or to change life style. Services that are "delivered" from the outside will have limited effect unless absorbed and taken over by the community. How long have physicians and nurses sat in health centres, seeing patients, and waiting for the health status of a population to improve? (In truth, those who so serve may not even ask questions about health status.)

Community participation is no less essential in dealing with the population growth—ecological deterioration complex. Personal and community decisions are at the heart of effective attacks on that set of problems. It takes little power of visualization to see herders and wood-gatherers, hunting far and wide for fodder or fuel, to appreciate how central their perceptions of problems are to any plan for solution.

Accordingly, services should relate to communities in at least the following ways:

in defining the problems — the community will be questioned and listened to, and, where possible will actually be involved in seeking information, as in community surveys. In the Aga Khan community-based programme in Kisumu, Kenya, communities carry out house-by-house surveys, analyse the data, and use the data in decision-making (*42*).

in decision-making — the community should be a party, even a leading party, in deciding what is to be done; this requires that the relevant information and issues requiring decisions be put forward in ways the community can understand; this is a key point in developing management information systems, where it is necessary to adjust the nature of the information to those who will make the decisions (*42*).

in financing — because the community is an essential partner in paying for health services; the possibility of governments being able to pay for health services is fast fading, and was probably illusory all along; importantly, only if the community is sharing in the costs does it gain the leverage whereby it might demand relevant and effective services (25).

Focus on the home and women

The role of women in effective implementation of PHC programmes must be seen as essential. The critical focus of most of PHC is the home, where families live in ways that are either healthy or burdened with risk, where behaviour is influenced by neighbours and family, and where decisions that affect health are made. The mother (and father) must have the knowledge, as well as the autonomy, to act as necessary to promote and protect health within the family.

Perhaps special points should be made about the education of women. There is no reason to hesitate over its importance, but we need to look beyond education as such if we are to appreciate the full importance of learning for the roles of women. First, it is too easy to equate education or literacy with knowledge, and to classifiy the illiterate as the problem. Secondly, education alone may not suffice to put the women in a position to take effective action. Some degree of autonomy or independence is required for them to make the decisions and take the actions necessary to promote improvements in health for themselves and their families (25).

There needs to be support that reaches to the home and family, such as:

- community health workers from the community, trained in the community, respected by the community, providing ready access to what they know and, when feasible, to the health services that back them up;
- family records including immunization status, growth monitoring chart, and information relating to risk factors in the mother and other family members;
- periodic surveillance visits at least by a supervised CHW, once every 1—3 months when children under two years are involved;
- clinical care for common problems and referral for more complex problems;
- sources of knowledge about the critical facts of family life.

Regarding knowledge relevant to family health, UNICEF points out that the most significant examples of social mobilization for development have been the spread of family planning and of the "green" revolution (43), though each of these programmes had some unintended negative consequences as well. Nevertheless, millions of families have been able to improve their own lives through the dissemination of available knowledge and affordable technologies. The same strategy is now being used with immunization and oral rehydration

47

therapy (ORT), and could be extended to other areas of knowledge related to maternal, child and family health.

The following is a listing of subject areas where a body of knowledge exists to which all families have a right (43):

— timing births;
— pregnancy;
— breast-feeding;
— promoting growth;
— immunization;
— diarrhoea;
— acute respiratory infection;
— home hygiene.

The father and family well-being

There is another issue that stands to be lost from sight as we focus so tightly on the mother and the children. It is the health of the father, and other members of the household. It is beyond argument that priority should go to mothers and children, but exclusive attention to them may not serve their best interests and, in any case, may not be supportive of the integrity of the family unit.

A man with active, infectious tuberculosis, or incapacitated with malaria, or with serious hypertension can threaten the well-being of his wife and children as surely as though they themselves were afflicted.

There is plentiful evidence that even the least developed countries are afflicted with mixtures of the diseases of poverty and the diseases of affluence. Attention should be given to analysis of the burdens of these disease patterns on families, and how different patterns should be handled so as to be supportive of the well-being of mothers and children, but also of the father and of the family as the critical social unit of the community. Risk factor analysis and the development of risk factor family profiles would be one approach.

There is something wrong with priorities when they call for such exclusive attention to one set of problems — those of women and children that — the result is either not noticing, or continually pushing away and out of sight, the matter of the family as a social unit whose health is critical to its integrity.

District-level support for the community

Support for the community from the district should include:

• supervision and on-going training of health workers who work in or reach out to communities;

• referral arrangements in which patients with urgent or complex problems can be referred to levels with the relevant competencies;

• involvement in discussions or communications whereby local concerns and ideas can be transmitted to higher levels of decision-making, so that communities are not cut off from central decisions that affect them;

- surveillance of health status and monitoring of programmes, possibly through continued reporting by CHWs, whereby the district level has accurate information about health conditions and concerns at community level.

Societies are made up of families and communities. Bureaucracies function at the margin of those social structures. Hopes for improvements in health reside with the families, not with technological packages, though technology has its part to play. Armed with knowledge of health, and related to health services they trust, families will do what they always do, act in their own best interests. Technology and management will be most effective and efficient when they connect directly with community structures and people and enlist their interest and commitment in dealing with the problems.

In the squatter settlements of Karachi, PHC programmes were stagnant in attempting to reduce infant mortality rates (the IMR was about 145 per 1000 live births in several field sites) until the community became involved and committed to dealing with the problems of malnutrition and diarrhoea. It was the mothers, supported by the CHWs, who made the effective attack on those problems.

Finally, it is shortsighted and misleading to expect and wait for government to answer the health problems of communities. Even if government has resources for health services, communities must still take a strong role, and where governmental services are weak or absent, the community must be self-reliant.

It should not be forgotten that people in the more developed societies are generally self-sufficient (though not always correct) in making decisions about their health, their behaviour, and where and when to seek health care. A reasonable goal in all societies is to promote self-reliance and reduce dependence.

Facilitating applications of science and technology in support of health for all

Science and its applications in technology form a two-edged sword for HFA. The capacity of science and technology to address problems is at the heart of modernization, and the potential for contributing to the development of even the poorest countries is very large. But science can be costly to pursue and apply, and the costs can be measured in terms of money, programmatic distortions, and human harm.

While much could be said about science and technology and their applications in the context of HFA, we will focus on five areas:

- evolution of biomedical science and applications to the Third World;
- the overriding problem of inadequate PHC infrastructures;

- indiscriminate transfers of technology;
- ethical implications of advances in technology;
- building a science base in the Third World.

Evolution of biomedical science and applications to the third world

Joshua Lederberg, Nobel Laureate and President of the Rockefeller University, describes three cycles or generations of biomedical science:[1]

> The first cycle, from Pasteur and Koch to about 1950, included the development of the germ theory of disease and the great advances in public health in the developed countries.

> The second cycle, from 1950 to about 1980, brought a profound understanding of cell biology of which DNA research was emblematic, as well as sophisticated advances in medical and surgical practice. What was less well understood and appreciated was how little these fundamental and applied branches of medicine related to one another.

> The third cycle began in about 1980, and is characterized not only by striking advances in biotechnology but also by a new convergence of DNA-oriented research with practical advances for such problems as schizophrenia, heart disease, diabetes, sickle cell anaemia and many others. A paradox is at work in which the most basic level of research generates understanding of fundamental disease processes that, in turn, allows practical steps of prevention or amelioration.

WHO's Advisory Committee on Medical Research (now the Advisory Committee on Health Research) recently assembled a group of eminent scientists to address the question: Which advances in the new biotechnologies are likely to have public health applications? The group identified a series of new concepts and techniques that are likely to have immediate as well as long-term results.[2] Lederberg's thesis of convergence of basic research and applications will be apparent in the following:

> - *Analysis of the structure and function of genomes of infectious agents to understand better the processes of infection and mechanisms of immunity.*

> WHO's Special Programme for Research and Training in Tropical Diseases, through its global network of collaborative research, has used basic techniques of immunology and recombinant DNA technology to achieve striking advances in understanding of the epidemiology, immunology and genetics of malaria. These advances bring us close, to having vaccines for malaria as well as to a much more penetrating understanding of the disease, which will be required when we encounter the inevitable limitations of immune protection.

---

[1] Bryant, J.H. *The evolution of equity in health — an examination of policies, programs and prospects for health for all in the Third World.* Presentation at the International Health Seminar Series, Washington, DC, 1983.

[2] *Report of the Advisory Committee on Medical Research to the Director-General, 1984.* Unpublished WHO document ACMR26/94.9 Report.

- *Identification of disease-specific heredity traits to provide a sound basis for genetic approaches of health promotion.*

  The total burden of genetic diseases in both developed and developing countries involves some 3—5% of the population. Sickle cell disease and thalassaemia, as examples, affect tens of millions of people. New methods for diagnosis of genetic abnormalities, including predictive tests and increasing understanding of the disease processes, offer changing approaches to management of these conditions.

- *Development of reliable and easy-to-use procedures for the diagnosis of communicable diseases.*

  Enzyme immunoassays, including notably the ELISAs (enzyme-linked immunosorbent assays), are used routinely to detect small amounts of constituents present in biological fluids or cells, and are adaptable to field use.

  Monoclonal antibodies have great potential for use in diagnostic assays including in simple field tests for the detection of antibodies as well as antigens.

There are also some relatively simple applications of science that have produced very practical technology for the Third World: cold-chain technology that helps ensure protection of vaccines against temperature extremes; oral rehydration therapy for diarrhoea, which is now pointing towards cereal-based solutions; diagnostic methods that can be applied in peripheral health centres, such as dip-stick and blotter paper tests; durable but accurate equipment, such as a battery-powered X-ray machine; microcomputers; a simple but reliable method for determining haemoglobin levels of blood; essential drugs, and country lists of generic drugs most appropriate to local therapeutic needs.

The overriding problem of inadequate PHC infrastructure
While we look to biomedical science for critical inputs towards solving some of the most intractable problems of Third World diseases, another set of problems stands at the front in terms of immediate priority — the weakness and general disarray of infrastructures for PHC.

The dominant problem of improving the health of people in the poorer countries is not lack of technology — it is inability to reach people with services. The technology is now in hand to reduce the great burdens of death and disease, but the service systems are not in place. While we will continue to applaud the efforts to advance science and to direct those efforts towards Third World problems, it is the strengthening of health service systems that holds the key to successful applications of science and technology. This calls attention to the importance of field-based research on health services development and on applications of technology within those health services.

Recently, in a remote desert area of Baluchistan (one of the provinces of Pakistan), I saw a young man and his family, all with active tuberculosis. Health services did not reach that corner of Asia, and, tragically, the family was dying of a diagnosable, preventable, curable disease.

While much of what goes into the development of PHC systems is known and applicable given local commitment and adequate resources, there remain serious gaps in knowledge and experience that need to be addressed through research. Whether or not to use community health workers, and how to use them, are matters of wide difference from country to country. Management information systems for tracking surveillance and guiding decisions is an emerging field. How to extend the PHC infrastructure to cover remote populations at very low cost is a complex question. What constitutes cost-effectiveness where the trade-off may be between cost and equity is an important question. Community-based approaches to financing health services are critical in an environment of declining resources. Local policy-makers need the guidance that research on such matters can provide.

Distortions from indiscriminate transfers of technology to the Third World

Advances in clinical medicine have added greatly to the diagnostic and therapeutic power of medicine, and immensely to its cost. A capacity to make decisions in the face of high and escalating costs is now an integral part of the management and practice of medical care, particularly in developed countries.

The complexity, sophistication and costs of diagnostic and therapeutic procedures have become so dominant as to push aside the more personal and humanly sensitive side of medical care. In the developed world, this is a matter of rising concern. In the Third World the problem borders on disaster. The transfer of technology has often been indiscriminate, the costs scandalous, and the technological distractions from priority needs ruinous. This is not to say that advancing technology must be excluded from the Third World, but sensitivity to needs and judgement about priority uses of resources must command first place.

But making decisions in this arena is complicated. Policy-makers and health professionals are, at best, trying to make sensible policy for long-term development, and so a dilemma develops between what is essential today and what is necessary as a base for tomorrow. Even familiar words add to the confusion: is excellence in health care to be defined in terms of sophistication of procedures, or in terms of equity? Obviously HFA would steer us towards equity as the guideline.

Professional self-interest enters the picture — one trained to use high technology equipment understandably wants to use it, and further his/her professional development, whether or not it is appropriate to local circumstances. And profit-making becomes a grim partner when commercial interests centre on selling technology rather than on facilitating balanced development.

Those who are advising or selling from the developed world have a difficult role. They are at their best when they help their partners to select judiciously from First World technology those things that are appropriate to transfer to Third World settings and budgets. They are at their worst when their own self-interests are narrow and they promote them.

It can also be difficult for the Third World decision-maker, if he/she is the only one in the local setting who is holding to equity as the dominant guiding principle.

Ethical implications of advances in technology

Equity, the conceptual heart of health for all, is fundamentally an ethical issue. Advances in technology can either promote or impede progress towards equity — promote, if oriented towards local needs with practical and low-cost applications; impede, if pointed towards problems of questionable importance without regard for the needs of general populations, practicality or cost.

Here are two edges of the technological sword. But many of the ethical issues that attend advances in technology are more subtle. They have to do with such questions as:

> The limits of therapy — how vigorously and for how long is this patient to be kept alive?

> The nature and uses of genetic information — do I have a right to know about my genetic self? Do I have a right not to know?

Entirely new questions may be precipitated by demographic shifts, technological advances and related escalations of costs. Even the seemingly straightforward meanings of "health" and "all" come into question:

> How do length of life and quality of life relate to the meaning and value of human life and therefore to the definition of "health" in health for all? Is there a genetic definition of a life worth living?

> Advances in the technology of genetic screening raise questions about the meaning of "all": with respect to my genetic self, is my responsibility to myself, my family or to succeeding generations? The concept of "all" in a genetic sense requires an intergenerational perspective.

> Consideration of acquired immunodeficiency syndrome (AIDS) draws attention to the risks of aggressive approaches to disease control in which afflicted persons whose cooperation is needed most become isolated beyond the reach of helping and being helped. New problems are seen in extending services to "all", including the alienated and the vulnerable.

Traditional professional, cultural and religious values may not provide clear guidance on such issues. It is at the level of policy-making that these questions are often most urgently addressed, yet policy-makers may have no more guidance on the issues than health professionals and lay persons.

The Council for International Organizations of Medical Sciences (CIOMS) and WHO have been addressing these issues through a series of conferences on health policy, ethics and human values. Together, these conferences have formed an international dialogue involving policy-makers, ethicists and health professionals from many countries, cultures, religions and political perspectives. The dialogue is attempting to address fundamental ethical issues that face policy-makers, with a particular concern for the ethical precepts that underly health for all (44).

Strengthening research capacities in Third World countries

Most problems of the Third World cannot be solved by technology transfer from the First World. They require solutions developed on the spot. But theory, method, and a spirit of inquiry — they come from science and form the basis for developing solutions locally. How is local capacity for dealing with problems to be strengthened? This is actually an old question, and the reason there is already a substantial science base in the Third World is because a number of those countries together with internationally oriented institutions have been working on this need for several decades.

For some problems of the Third World, the research strengths are in the Third World; for others the lead is in the developed world. In either case, close and continued interaction between scientists is imperative — intellectual dialogue and exchange of methods and materials is the life blood of science.

A time-tested approach is to link Third World scientists and their institutions with counterparts in the developed world. More and more centres of scientific research are becoming established in the Third World, and they will be able to serve as points of linkage with other Third World scientists in some fields. What is needed, and is under way, though to a more limited extent than is desirable, is training in science and its applications.

A problem of increasing seriousness is that the cost of training in the developed countries is rising rapidly at the same time that resources in the Third World are diminishing. Ideally, the training would all take place close to home in the country or region. A now historic example of this kind of development was the Rockefeller Foundation's long-term support of Mahidol University in Thailand, which resulted in a strong centre for master's and doctoral level biomedical research and training. Currently, the WHO/World Bank/UNDP Special Programme for Research and Training in Tropical Diseases, in collaboration with other funding agencies, invests substantial resources in individual and institutional capacity building for research.

Lacking local capacity for advanced research training, at least the first stages should take place in one's own country or region, say to the master's level or its equivalent, and the "topping off", say for advanced research experience and possibly an advanced degree, could be done in a developed country institution. But this approach should be seen as an interim measure, on the way to enhancement of Third World universities.

An endless list of interesting and important research subjects could be offered, but one will be emphasized here — district health services. Using a district as a research field site will allow a broad range of questions to be asked — equity, coverage, management, manpower, community roles, risk factors in relation to maternal mortality, programme effectiveness, diagnostic technologies, disease control methods, cost and benefit. Here, too, collaborative approaches with other sectors could be developed to focus not only on district health problems but also on the broader issues of population growth and ecosystem instability.

Developing leadership for health for all

Leadership for HFA is there, but in short supply. There is the issue. Is it possible to achieve a major shift, in which those who can assume such leadership positions become dominant, rather than occasional? Numbers are important. HFA, at its core, is a value issue. But the problems it addresses are largely quantitative — all people, not some. Equity, not inequity. All children will be monitored, not some. Rates. Numbers. HFA must be quantitatively effective. The number of people who assume leadership roles for HFA must be quantitatively significant. Their influence must be pervasive.

Here, we will deal with selected aspects of this problem:

- leadership development for HFA;
- promoting greater effectiveness in health manpower development;
- the uses of PHC field sites for leadership preparation;
- dilemmas that face universities in their efforts to implement their most easily stated and most laudable objectives.

WHO and leadership development

WHO has undertaken a major effort to identify and promote leadership for HFA. A series of regional and interregional meetings with leaders from various countries, fields and levels of expertise, has led to the preparation of materials to assist in enhancing leadership capacities, and the theme of the Technical Discussions held during the World Health Assembly in May 1988 was Leadership Development for HFA (see page 104).

The process WHO is following is most unusual: the meetings are structured for informal dialogue, calling on actual leaders to use their insights and experience to identify their own characteristics and the critical factors involved in the development and utilization of such leadership. These are shared among leaders and those with leadership potential. The possibility that this process can become self-generating is intriguing. That depends, in the first instance, on how many people believe that HFA is worth this kind of attention and introspection. In that sense, it is a test of HFA, as well as a process that could contribute to HFA.

Promoting greater effectiveness
in health manpower development

WHO, rightly, emphasizes close relationships between health manpower preparation and health services development, which it terms health systems and manpower development — HSMD (45).

Bringing that integration to reality is difficult, if not impossible, in countries where the education of health personnel is entirely separate from their deployment and management in health services. When one proceeds independently of the other, dysfunctional results are inevitable. Surely the most flagrant example is that of medical schools increasing enrolments without reference to national manpower development strategies, resulting in ludicrous surpluses of manpower that will require 40 years to redress. In 1986, WHO and CIOMS held a conference entitled Health Manpower Out of Balance, which dealt with those issues (46).

Another set of manpower development issues that claims much of WHO's attention centres on increasing both the quality and relevance of the education of health personnel. The words that form the objectives read like an exercise in hyphenation:

A. problem-oriented
    student-oriented
    self-learning
    life-long learning

B. competency-based
    community-based
    multi-professional (team-focused)
    multi-sectoral.

It would be a mistake, however, to dismiss these expressions as simply jargon or "WHO-ese". Each expression, in fact, represents a move from a traditional focus of thinking and action to the broader interactions required for effective functioning in PHC settings. Every hyphen takes us another step away from the isolation of traditional educational approaches of individual professions. These compound words fall into two groups, one having to do with methodologies for teaching and learning (A); the other with relevance and effectiveness with respect to health services (B).

These concepts have been the centre of interest of the Network of Community-Oriented Educational Institutions for Health Sciences, the secretariat of which is located at the University of Limburg, Maastricht, Netherlands. This international network includes thus far about 50 universities with a commitment to the above-mentioned concepts. It is probably accurate to say that the members who come from the developed world are more effective in dealing with the first group of concepts, while those from the developing world concentrate more on the second group. It is of considerable interest that as the Network has pursued the two sets of objectives, they have identified the principles of HFA as their major guide in developing educational programmes and methods to ensure the relevance of education to function. Here, then, is an international mechanism to promote improvements in the quality and relevance of the education of health personnel.

Unfortunately, this progressive approach to health manpower development is not widespread among universities. Indeed, many are simply aloof from efforts to extend services to the underserved, they scoff at subjects that carry the terminology of prevention and equity, and are more centres of scepticism and cynicism about HFA than points for sparking leadership to deal with national problems. Of course, the reasons will be clothed in acceptable terminology having to do with clinical excellence and science-based medicine. One could wish that such institutions were in the minority and hope that their numbers would be diminishing. Constructive action and movement into leadership roles are sorely needed from the universities.

The question remains, how is it possible to develop programmes that respect the hyphens? It is possible, of course, but there are some guiding rules. The experience of the Aga Khan University, Karachi, as a new institution trying to develop some of these approaches, may be helpful.

Using PHC field sites for leadership preparation

At the Aga Khan University in Pakistan, we consider that the community-based PHC systems we have developed as a basis for our educational programmes for doctors and nurses are absolutely essential. The first step is to bring doctors and nurses into leadership positions in the field sites. For PHC to be effective, those in the leadership roles must have the relevant competencies, they must work in a multi-professional setting with other personnel in a team, and they must be sensitive to the need for multisectoral action. When they do not have the appropriate competencies, when they do not work together as a team, the PHC systems either stagnate or fall apart.

Thus our medical and nursing students are brought into such settings, where they work together in the field under the guidance of those teams of personnel. Without functioning PHC programmes, and without role models in place, as was the case earlier in the development of the university, the ideas behind the hyphenated words become more theory than substance. Now, these ideas live in practice — not always shaped as one would like, not always effective, but the faults are visible and correcting them becomes part of the process of teaching and learning.

Without such functioning PHC systems that embody the objectives of the teaching programme, one is left with theory, simulations, role-playing. Institutions that can actually develop community-based PHC programmes and use them as sites for teaching have a strong advantage. Not to develop such field programmes is to risk theorizing alone and drifting towards irrelevance. The thesis that "those who teach should serve, and those who serve should teach" (45), is more than academic poetry; it is at the heart of maintaining relevance between education and function.

A word about nursing education in this context. Without nursing leadership on the PHC team, we would have no team. The community health nurse plays a pivotal role in training and supervising middle-level and community health workers and in relating their work to the oversight of the community health doctor. She or he plays a critical role in guiding the effort of the PHC team to deal with the problems of women and development, as in enabling women to cope with risks to health in the home environment. WHO has emphasized these issues in the training of nurse teachers and managers, particularly through post-basic educational programmes (47). We are fortunate in having a strong community health component in the basic nursing educational programme, and will continue that emphasis in post-basic programmes as well.

Continuing education of health personnel is scarcely present in the Third World, yet no one would support the notion that basic education is sufficient for coping with the complexities of health in a changing world. Again, the value of a functioning and demonstrably effective community-based PHC

57

system for educational purposes is beyond question. And, given the facts that the PHC system is community-based, multiprofessional, multisectoral, and problem-oriented, its use for teaching and learning for all types of personnel — doctors, nurses, managers, middle-level workers, community workers, and for teachers to continue to learn — is quite natural.

Finally, the field programmes can be expanded to include district health systems, which would incorporate front-line hospitals, so that students and health teams are involved in the full spectrum of services from community-based PHC, to support from hospitals of a PHC network, to districtwide management of a health system, to intersectoral action on development problems. Here, the concept of a health team is expanded to include the different members and functions of teams at different levels of the system.

Notice how far these arrangements extend beyond the traditional relationship between the university and its teaching hospital. They require the university to be associated with multiple components of a health services system. Instead of a university and its teaching hospital we have a university and its teaching health system.

A health-for-all university? Some dilemmas
The Aga Khan University (AKU) in Karachi is approaching the concept of a health-for-all university. In doing so, it has encountered a series of critical questions, some of which would carry it beyond the usual responsibilities and purposes of a university.

First, a brief background for staging these key questions. AKU is the first private university in Pakistan, chartered by the government and functioning under the aegis of the Pakistan Medical and Dental Council. While privately funded, most of its field activities are financed through international granting sources.

The university's central objective is to contribute to improvements in the health of the people of Pakistan. The Department of Community Health Sciences has the lead in implementing that objective, with vigorous cooperation from other departments. In keeping with that objective, the university intends:

> to train young doctors and nurses for leadership in dealing with the health and development problems of Pakistan, particularly in the more deprived communities;

> to develop field programmes in which the typical problems of the country can be addressed through health systems based on PHC.

To be very brief:

> The university has allocated 20% of curriculum time in each year of study to community health sciences, and has developed a community-based curriculum in which students spend substantial time in communities; each class of students is associated with the same community for five years.

The university has developed community-based PHC systems in a series of urban and rural field sites.

The urban PHC programmes have taken the form of prototypes of PHC that meet the principles of HFA — universal coverage and care according to need; community involvement; information systems for monitoring and evaluation; effectiveness in improving health status indicators; some cross-sectoral activity; and affordability in terms of local resources. A cluster of five such sites forms the urban equivalent of a district. These programmes have been developed in close cooperation with the urban government.

In a rural district, the university is collaborating with the provincial government to improve district health services including districtwide management.

In the high mountains of the north of Pakistan, the university is collaborating with the Aga Khan Health Services of Pakistan (a nongovernmental organization) and government in attempting to develop methods of extending health services throughout that remote and difficult terrain.

An Advisory Council on Health Policy Research involving government and AKU, among others, is being set up to facilitate consideration of health policy issues that warrant research.

Now to the critical questions:

The traditional responsibilities of universities include education, research, and service. AKU has developed HFA prototypes of PHC to facilitate education and research. *Does the responsibility of the university extend to designing and testing prototypes so that they might be replicated by government and other NGOs?* In our judgement that is an appropriate role for the university.

While the leadership of health services in Pakistan is highly competent and committed, implementation at local levels, particularly in the large poor urban conglomerates, is often very problematic. Realistically, the prototypes will probably not be replicated in those settings unless the university becomes directly involved. *Should the university's responsibilities extend to assisting in the wide-scale implementation of HFA prototypes of PHC?* Our university is examining this question carefully: special concerns are directed towards competing needs of the university, such as the teaching programme; towards the time and energy availability of current leaders; and towards short- and long-term resource considerations (*48*).

Our educational programmes appear to have some promise for turning out young people who will be both competent and willing to deal with the most pressing problems of the country, either at the community level, or at the district (or comparable) level, such as in front-line hospitals, where they would be involved in backing up community-based PHC systems. A current problem, however, is that the health services are not functioning at a level of effectiveness that makes the relevant positions attractive for medical and nursing graduates. As in so many countries, lacking interesting opportunities to use what they have learned, they might be expected to turn in other directions.

What can the university do about this dilemma? The university might join with government and other parties in replicating useful prototypes and in improving existing health services settings. A network of such field sites could be put together for placement of graduates. Possibly the graduates could join a programme rather than simply being assigned to a distant site — an HFA service corps? — with potential for on-going professional enrichment and career development. In short, *should the university become operationally involved in improving health services, including establishing placement opportunities for its graduates, in order to ensure opportunities for them to progress into leadership roles?* Here again, the university is looking at such options carefully.

These questions raise issues that are very profound for universities. They place universities in a classical quandary:

to remain in the cloister and protect their capacity for education and research, but risk isolation from societal realities;

to go out and deal with societal realities, grapple with the problems as they exist, but risk being engulfed and destabilized by them (not a trivial problem in Third World countries).

There is a middle ground, and these questions are part of the search for it. What is clear and underlies the examination of these dilemmas is that institutional objectives so easy to state, so important to put forward — such as to produce leaders and contribute to improvement of health services — may remain unrealized unless the university moves beyond its traditional ground, in order to become operationally involved in establishing those leadership roles and in implementing those services.

Here is another example of the need to consider new ways of analysing problems, and new mechanisms, partners and resources in dealing with them.

What does HFA ask of us? Where does wisdom lie?

Dr Mahler's eight questions asked at Alma-Ata

At Alma-Ata in 1978, Dr Mahler said that it was important to reach agreement on the principles of PHC and on the action that will have to be taken by countries and at international level to ensure that it is properly understood and that it is systematically introduced or strengthened throughout the world, so that it becomes a living reality whose implementation no reactionary forces in the health world will ever be able to stop.

He then asked eight questions, which are reproduced opposite.

(1) Are you ready to address yourselves seriously to the existing gap between the health "haves" and the health "have nots" and to adopt concrete measures to reduce it?

(2) Are you ready to ensure the proper planning and implementation of primary health care in coordinated efforts with other relevant sectors, in order to promote health as an indispensable contribution to the improvement of the quality of life of every individual, family and community as part of overall socioeconomic development?

(3) Are you ready to make preferential allocations of health resources to the social periphery as an absolute priority?

(4) Are you ready to mobilize and enlighten individuals, families and communities in order to ensure their full identification with primary health care, their participation in its planning and management and their contribution to its application?

(5) Are you ready to introduce the reforms required to ensure the availability of relevant manpower and technology, sufficient to cover the whole country with primary health care within the next two decades at a cost you can afford?

(6) Are you ready to introduce, if necessary, radical changes in the existing health delivery system so that it properly supports primary health care as the overriding health priority?

(7) Are you ready to fight the political and technical battles required to overcome any social and economic obstacles and professional resistance to the universal introduction of primary health care?

(8) Are you ready to make unequivocal political commitments to adopt primary health care and to mobilize international solidarity to attain the objective of health for all by the year 2000?

The Director-General's remarks were highly appropriate and seriously challenging at Alma-Ata, as those of us who were there remember. But perhaps the most interesting thing that can be said about them now is that while they were precisely the right questions to ask in 1978, they are, possibly without change, also the right questions to ask in 1988.

Those questions were asked by the Director-General at a time of setting up an entirely different kind of institutional programme for WHO, and represented a deliberate probing at the understanding, readiness and toughness of the Member States to undertake what he saw with remarkable foresight would have to be done.

Now, a decade later, we have renewed conviction that HFA has the social, moral, political and technical strength to serve as an effective international guideline for the coming decade. But this time the lines are more clearly drawn. Some battles have been won, some have been lost, and the most difficult ones still lie ahead. There are veterans who know the way, and new leaders ready to join in. The tasks ahead may be all the more difficult because of the passing of time.

Given the hardened agenda that must be put forward in the face of nearly intractable problems, the Director-General's questions are still the right questions. We must still probe at the understanding, readiness and toughness of the Member States to undertake what remains to be done.

Conclusions

As WHO turns the corner of the first decade after Alma-Ata, it needs to ready itself to face a new set of problems. In particular, it must appreciate that tomorrow will not be yesterday, and that yesterday's answers, though they brought glory, will not serve tomorrow.

I. Health for all — a living reality

Ten years since Alma-Ata.
It is now clear that the concepts and principles of HFA formulated by the World Health Assembly in 1977 and elaborated at Alma-Ata in 1978 provided the world with ethical precepts, political imperatives and technical directions that have since become critical guidance to the health and development community worldwide.

Of course, not all have heard, and not all have seen what was meant by the idea of HFA. That is not surprising. Scepticism is not a rare commodity, and it has its uses. What has been surprising is how widely HFA has been accepted and used, in whole or in part, by health policy-makers, programme planners, funding organizations, politicians, health personnel, schoolteachers, newspaper reporters, professors, mothers, schoolchildren.

A further surprise is how influential it has been in the policies and programmes of the *developed countries,* given the initial concern that the more affluent part of the world would consider HFA as applying to poor countries only. In fact, HFA has become not only a basis for national health strategies of WHO — that might be expected — but also a basis for national health strategies of many of the developed Member States. That is not to say that there are not serious problems to be overcome, particularly in view of burgeoning clinical technology, rising costs and depersonalization of medical care.

Less surprising, but no less gratifying, has been the general acceptance of the HFA strategy by the poorer countries in formulating their national and regional strategies. Here is the acid test of HFA. Given a commitment to equity, and a priority to the poor, can the precepts, commitments, structures and resources guided by or generated by HFA make a difference in the health and well-being of the poor of the world? We will return to that question.

Scepticism, contrary belief, disdain — these have their place in social, scientific and political discourse, particularly if bolstered with constructive challenge and alternative proposals. The subject is too important, however, to be thrown aside in contempt, and there is some of that.

Overall, HFA has survived and spread because it both draws on and contributes to four important fields of thinking and action — ethical, political, social and technical. If any of these four elements was removed, it would be seriously damaging to HFA in concept and implementation.

At Alma-Ata Dr Mahler said that it was necessary that HFA be properly understood and systematically strengthened throughout the world ... *"so that it becomes a living reality whose implementation no reactionary forces in the health world will ever be able to stop"*. It now seems highly likely that what Dr Mahler wanted in 1978 is well on the way in 1988.

There was never a thought, of course, that HFA meant that the world would be free of health problems. There are and will always be serious and unresolved problems. A purpose of HFA is to provide a conceptual framework for thinking about that multiplicity of problems and for guiding decisions about priorities and action. One of the very constructive outcomes of WHO's work with HFA has been the development of monitoring and reporting procedures through which WHO and the countries can follow trends in health-related problems, including progress, or lack of it, toward HFA targets, and for planning accordingly.

II. Health for all — beyond the year 2000

The quest for HFA will not end in the year 2000, or in the year 2100. No country can solve all of its health problems, and new problems continue to emerge in every country. These are biological and social realities of life. The goal of the year 2000 nevertheless continues to be a milestone of great significance. Associated with it are imperatives that identified targets be met in every country, with particular emphasis on reductions in mortality and morbidity in the poorest countries.

At the same time, we need to look over the horizon, beyond the turn of the century to the problems of that time, some continuing from the present, others emerging entirely new. The capacity for dealing with those problems, in that era, is being built now, and will be strengthened further between now and the year 2000. Indeed, it is likely that an extremely important long-term contribution of the current HFA movement will be to establish in every country, in every community, an evolving capacity to deal with health problems that arise.

Thus, the goal of HFA remains unchanging, but the targets will shift, from those suited to the decade preceding the year 2000, to those relevant to future times and places. Key principles will remain — equity, effectiveness, affordability, community involvement. Problems will change, as will the technologies and social and organizational mechanisms to grapple with them. **Here, at the midpoint between Alma-Ata and the year 2000, our goals should be:**

- **to identify the critical challenges to be met between now and the turn of the century, and to show that headway can be made against the most solution-resistant problems;**

- **to lay the groundwork for the continuing efforts that must follow the turn of the century, that will lead to appropriate changes of strategy necessary to consolidate the pursuit of HFA beyond the year 2000.**

III. The health haves and the health have-nots

At Alma-Ata, Dr Mahler asked: "Are you ready to address yourself seriously to the existing gap between the health "haves" and the health "have-nots" and to adopt concrete measures to reduce it?"

What emerges clearly in 1988 is the global dichotomy of the health "haves" and the health "have-nots". Of course, it does not divide neatly; there is a spectrum with countries strung along the gradient from poorest to richest, from highest under-fives mortality rates to the lowest — but there is a key point to be made. It has to do with a country's capacity for coping with its health and development problems.

Many countries are moving along the gradient at a pace measurable with familiar indicators: as per capita income increases, as literacy increases, under-five mortality rate and maternal mortality rate decrease, and so forth. There is a rough predictability about the process, though there are many exceptions in which countries are moving either more rapidly or more slowly in health than would be expected from socioeconomic levels, and we learn from these exceptions (25).

On page 20 we discussed the use of some statistical indicators of health development and the slowness with which they have changed. Here, we can make two points:

- the slowness represents a continuing burden of suffering and death that should be considered totally unacceptable, and calls for urgent attention;

- the slowness may be stagnation, an entrapment in a development reversal from which the countries concerned are unable to extricate themselves; the signals are less clear here, but that is all the more reason for urgent attention.

IV. The hand for the poor

WHO has a constitutional mandate to concern itself with the health problems of all countries of the world, but that has never kept it from giving special attention to its greatest concerns. One talent of that socially sensitive bureaucracy is that it has managed to give attention to all problems considered worthy of mention by Member States and the public while not losing sight of either genuine threats to the world's health or the deepest needs of the destitute and vulnerable of the world.

In one sense, WHO's concern for the poor is above priorities. Priorities have to do with choices. WHO has moved beyond such choices — by virtue of its own internal ethic it has permanently committed itself to serving the poor. It takes care of the world with one hand, and of the poor with the other. We have something to say about what is done with the hand that reaches to the poor.

We go back to the two points made above about slowness of progress in health and development, and along those lines define two sets of problems.

One set of problems is best depicted by the very high maternal and under-five mortality rates mentioned on page 20. The reasons for these extremely high death rates are generally known and widely discussed and written about. There is still much to be learned, and local differences in causes and approaches are critically important. None the less, there are reasonably well understood approaches to dealing with them, largely through well organized and managed health services that are supportive of PHC with strong and meaningful community involvement, linked in turn with other sectors of development.

Key points here are that while our knowledge is not complete, it is substantial; and while there are many problems of implementation, we are familiar with the terrain on which those problems need to be worked out. Global, regional and national expertise, and networks, have been working on these problems. The global health machinery is tuned to these problems.

The further point needs to be made, however, that the problems we are speaking of are solution-resistant. The global health machinery in its current state is not adequate. Progress has been slow despite growing understanding of the problems, and despite progress in health system development and emergence of new technologies. It would be a serious mistake for WHO to believe it could solve these problems with more of the same. The persistence of the problems is saying something to us, if we have ears to hear — what is being done is not enough.

The second set of problems has to do with *the interaction of population growth and ecosystem instability*, a form of "development-gone-wrong". In the classical demographic transition, high birth rates and high death rates proceed into the transitional stage in which death rates come down but not birth rates and population growth rates increase; the transition is completed when birth rates are brought down, and population growth rates decrease as well.

Things go wrong when countries get trapped in the middle or second stage — excessive and prolonged population growth leads to severe ecological and economic consequences. Fragile ecosystems cannot carry indefinitely increasing population burdens, agricultural productivity diminishes, incomes fall, landlessness increases, rural populations migrate to urban centres, social and political instabilities ensue. Rising morbidity and mortality are integral to these ecological and economic disasters (*30*).

65

Some Third World nations are becoming entrapped in this second stage — they cannot complete the demographic transition, they are caught, unable to put together the social, economic, agricultural and health strategies and programmes that will help them escape. The full seriousness of this problem remains to be determined, but the possibility must be kept open that they may have missed the opportunity to complete the transition; that they face the grim alternative of returning to the first stage of continuing high death rates as well as high birth rates.

This second set of problems contrasts sharply with the first (although they may overlap to a considerable degree); it calls for different responses. Here, experience is more limited. Though there have been extensive studies of aspects of this problem, much of the experience is recent. The knowledge base is thin, and research will be essential, but there is limited experience with where and how the research should be done. The problem as a whole does not fall clearly into one disciplinary domain or another. Multidisciplinarity is obviously necessary. Health problems, including those related to fertility, are embedded in the others, and the health sector will have a crucial role to play, but it must be played as part of the larger development.

To address this set of problems, WHO will need to go on to new ground. The global health machinery in its current form is even less ready for this set of problems than for the first. But one of WHO's strengths has been its willingness and ability to change direction and pace as required by the problems.

V. New directions, new partnerships, new mechanisms, new resources

These two sets of problems — high maternal and under-five mortality rates and population growth/ecosystem instability — test our thinking about WHO's current and future capabilities and strategies. What do they tell us?

- First, that these are serious problems afflicting the poor and most vulnerable of the world, and that WHO must respond to their needs.

- Secondly, that these are especially difficult problems. In the first instance, even though the content is familiar, they will have to be addressed in solution-resistant settings, with special attention to conditions of extreme underdevelopment. In the second instance, the problems are of a new kind, involving new scientific questions, requiring extensive intersectoral collaboration. Health is at or close to the centre but in new contexts of development-gone-wrong.

- Third, dealing with these problems will require fresh responses from WHO: new ways of analysing problems, new types of expertise, new organizational structures, new mechanisms for interacting with other parties and with the problems, new resources and uses of resources, and new scales of action.

As WHO turns the corner of the first decade after Alma-Ata, it needs to ready itself to face a new set of problems. In particular, it must appreciate that tomorrow will not be yesterday, and that yesterday's answers, though they brought glory, will not serve tomorrow.

These two problem sets also offer up challenges in each of the five areas of concern that we consider critical avenues for addressing the broad health problems of the poorest countries. The key ideas in these five areas are summarized below.

VI. Strengthening political and social interventions

Political commitment is a clear prerequisite to progress towards HFA, but by itself does not carry a country very far along the road to HFA. Policies, budgetary allocations, organizational rearrangements, assignment of strong leaders to key posts, and continuous support for PHC at the district level and beyond are critical ingredients.

Countries are coming to know more clearly the full range of interacting factors required for effective health services, and how crucial is their integration. A critical role for WHO is to continue to bring visibility to these factors and interactions so that at the country level they cannot be side-stepped.

A problem largely beyond the control or influence of individual countries is the ice-cold climate for development support. Perspectives that centre on materialism rather than equity; on narrow views of economic development rather than longer-term needs for social development; lack of understanding of or confidence in the processes of development, or even outright contempt for the people in developing countries, find their ways into development policies. Some of these are aggravated during times of recession, as in the downturn of the world economy in the early 1980s.

The recession of 1980—83 led to extraordinary debt burdens on the developing countries, which in turn led to the need for major economic "adjustments". Adjustment policies frequently contributed to severe worsening of conditions among vulnerable groups, including deterioration in health status. While there is increasing recognition of the negative effects of such adjustment policies, this is indicative of how health and other aspects of development fall victim to shifts in economic policy that focus narrowly on economic as opposed to broader aspects of social development.

A strong agenda for HFA to the end of the century makes social and political action imperative. Ways must be found to enlist the participation of the wide variety of literally thousands of potentially interested parties — NGOs, including particularly those that are indigenous to the Third World: universities; industry; community organizations; student groups; and individual citizens, many of whom are waiting for indications of useful directions in which to apply their resources and energies.

VII. Strengthening district health systems based on primary health care

District health systems based on PHC are at the centre of the HFA effort. Unfortunately, such systems are often weak, with little or no impact on the health of the population. Two particular deficiencies may be mentioned here.

One is an inability and even lack of interest in measuring health status, through morbidity rates, for example, or other indicators that would define the existing problems and provide a basis for evaluating programme effectiveness. The combination of lack of evaluative data and lack of placement of accountability results in systems that are blind to their own effectiveness, or lack of it, and powerless to correct drift or failure.

The other is the problem of manpower deficiencies. On the one hand are the irrelevance and ineffectiveness of much of the educational preparation received by health workers, who often lack the competencies required for the work that has to be done. On the other hand is the lack of support given by the health services to health workers; the neglect of their needs and unresponsiveness to their requests is consistent, widespread and destructive of their potential for effectiveness.

Despite these problems, there is immense potential for district health systems based on PHC being able to progress towards HFA. The world is learning how to develop more effective systems, supportive of community involvement in health activities, with health personnel who are well trained, motivated and supported in their field settings, and with management information systems that can support monitoring and evaluation. The distance between the current reality and what is a reasonable expectation is narrowing.

WHO's programme for strengthening district health systems is an important initiative, particularly as it seeks to enlist the collaboration of a number of rural and urban districts in the Third World which will be able to provide vital lessons from on-going activities for collaborating partners. Three areas of major importance are continuously evolving in the district context:

- preparation of health personnel for effective functioning in district programmes and their continuing education and support in the field;
- management technologies including planning, financial management, and health information systems, including the appropriate use of microcomputers;
- social and technical interactions with communities, with increasing shifts of responsibility and authority for decisions to community people, particularly in a cross-sectoral context.

Focusing on district health systems in relation to PHC provides an essential mechanism for probing at the factors that bear on difficult problem areas such as maternal and child mortality and the interactions of population growth and ecological deterioration.

Further emphasis needs to be given to enlisting others — universities, international organizations, ministries of health — to turn greater attention to the district as the geopolitical unit that is generally well suited to working through the more complex problems of health and development.

VIII. Supporting community-based and home-based health activities

It appears that the community may be moving to the centre of the development stage. That possibility is still fragile, and may represent wishful thinking, but the combination of increasing understanding from government ministries and from international organizations, plus the power people take on to themselves through the political process, at least give us exciting examples.

As mentioned on page 47, the role of women in the implementation of PHC programmes must be seen as essential. A major requirement of the health services is to provide the basic knowledge needed by families to act responsibly in taking care of themselves. For them not to have such knowledge leads to both dependence and ignorance, neither of which has a place in community development.

In addition, some attention to the health of family members other than mothers and young children, as through risk factor assessment, may also serve the interests of the mother and children as well as supporting the integrity of the family unit.

There is also growing understanding that governments cannot cover the costs of health services in anything approaching their entirety. Communities must increasingly share in those costs, or be left either without care or without a say in the kind of care that will be given.

IX. Science and technology in support of HFA

Science has much to offer to HFA, and in some areas the most advanced scientific insight and methodologies are needed almost on an emergency scale, as in grappling with the problem of AIDS. There are other calls on science, some less dramatic, but no less important. There are, for example, new applications of diagnostic methods that can be used at the periphery of health services. New vaccines will add importantly to the armamentarium of immunizations.

But there is a point to be made about technology and health services systems. It is probably accurate to say that the most serious deficiencies in improving health in the Third World that relate to science, do not have to do with the shortage of technology, but with inadequacies of infrastructures of health services that could bring the benefits of technology to the people.

Distortions can also occur as a result of the indiscriminate transfer of technology from the First to the Third World. The leading problem created by such transfers is the diversion of budget and attention from problems that can be addressed at the PHC level. In times of great fiscal constraint, competition between the transfer of advanced technology and the needs of PHC will become stronger, and the need for decision-making strength oriented towards equity will be very great. Advances in technology also raise ethical questions for which traditional, professional, cultural and religious values may not provide guidance.

Most problems of the Third World cannot be solved by technology transfer from the First World. They require solutions developed on the spot, and capacity-building in research is essential. The strategy for accomplishing that task must be based on detailed knowledge of current research capacities in the Third World as well as a sound understanding of how research is done and how people are helped to become proficient at it. This is an ideal enterprise for North—South collaboration that builds on established experience in this field. Emerging needs for enhanced research capacity must be addressed in the context of extreme resource constraints and the search begun for new resources, new mechanisms, and new partners.

X. Leadership for health for all

Without effective leadership, HFA will founder. The question is, how is leadership directed toward HFA to be found, developed and enhanced? WHO has embarked on an imaginative approach to the study and promotion of leadership development, the subject of the Technical Discussions held during the Forty-first World Health Assembly in May 1988.

There is a paradox about leadership in the Third World. Formally trained and experienced leaders are in short supply, and often over-used. At the same time, there are vast numbers with leadership potential who are untrained and inexperienced. There is much to be done, therefore, in supporting those in leadership roles, often few in number, while at the same time establishing opportunities for training and experience for others. Additionally, new paths for advancement of leaders, both trained and untrained, can be created to avoid dead ends in job or career development.

The cornerstone of WHO's approach to manpower development is its integration with health services development, thus health systems and manpower development, or HSMD. Parallel emphases focus on strengthening educational methodologies, as in problem-oriented, student-oriented, self-learning, and also on relevance to health services, as in competency-based, community-based, team-focused learning experiences. These terms are more than academic jargon; they represent key ideas in the interaction between education and function. Operational PHC programmes, in a community or a district, provide ideal locations for conceptualizing and implementing such educational programmes.

Universities have a critical role to play in leadership development in the health sector, particularly in preparing personnel to develop and lead more effective health services. Curiously, however, there are serious questions as to whether many universities can or even want to play that role. Is it not odd to have to put it that way? The responsibility for producing leaders is one of the primary responsibilities societies have given to universities, yet in the health sector, there is a distinct lack of confidence that many can or will do so. This may have to do with disdain for the concept of HFA, but is probably deeper, arising from conflicts of purpose between pursuing advances in medical science and responding to social needs, and how universities make institutional choices. Whatever the cause, it is an issue that needs to be better understood.

Finally, we return to the Director-General's remarks at Alma-Ata in 1978. Can we build an agreement and an understanding of HFA that will make it a living reality? The answer in 1988 is that we appear to be well on the way to that accomplishment. And having health for all as a living reality, we must use it well, for the poor, and for the world.

Alma-Ata reaffirmed at Riga

A statement of renewed and strengthened commitment to health for all by the year 2000 and beyond, adopted at the WHO meeting "From Alma-Ata to the year 2000: a midpoint perspective", Riga, USSR, 22–25 March 1988.

Preface

The meeting in Riga, USSR, from 22 to 25 March 1988, brought together experts from all WHO regions as well as representatives of UNICEF, UNDP and nongovernmental organizations.

The participants concluded that the health for all concept has made strong positive contributions to the health and well-being of people in all nations. Nevertheless, they noted that problems remain which call for increased commitment and action to ensure more effective implementation of primary health care.

They strongly reaffirmed the Declaration of Alma-Ata and called for the principles and spirit of health for all to be made a permanent goal by all countries.

Introduction to the actions at Riga

At the International Conference on Primary Health Care held in Alma-Ata in 1978, the nations of the world joined together in expressing the need for urgent action by all governments, all health and development workers, and the world community to protect and promote the health of all the people of the world.

These concerns, expressed at the World Health Assembly in 1977, were emphasized again in the Declaration of Alma-Ata which stated: that a main social target should be the attainment by all people of the world by the year 2000 of a level of health that will permit them to lead a socially and economically productive life; and that primary health care is the key to attaining this target as part of development in the spirit of social justice. It was also stated that health, peace and development are intimately related to one another, and that each must be pursued and protected in the interests of the well-being of mankind.

The experiences of the Member States in health development over the ten years since the Alma-Ata conference make it clear that the concepts and principles of health for all have provided the world with moral, political, social and technical guidance that has enabled countries to deal forthrightly with the problems of inequity in health care and the ill health of their populations.

This period has also demonstrated the potential importance of political action in contributing to health for all, such as action to decrease military confrontations and reduce defence expenditure, improve trade and economic relations, and the efforts to help resolve the problems of external debt.

Most countries have made considerable gains in increasing the equity and effectiveness of health services and in improving the health and well-being of their populations, thus affirming the validity and strategies of WHO's goal of health for all. Some striking examples can be given of improvements in coverage, effectiveness and quality of programmes:

- Immunization rates in most countries of the world have increased from about 5% of children in developing countries in 1970, to more than 50% in the late 1980s.

- Decreasing infant, under-five and maternal mortality rates are evidence of remarkable progress; in many countries, under-five mortality rates have decreased by more than 50% since 1950.

- Many countries have based their national health policies on the concepts of health for all, emphasizing health promotion, including improvements in life-styles, and decentralizing initiative to districts, cities and local communities.

Despite widespread progress, it is evident that the gains have not been uniform, either between countries or within them. All countries recognize the need perpetually to fight against ill health even though the nature of health problems will change. Looking ahead to the turn of the century and beyond, it is clear that maintaining health and ensuring equity must be a permanent goal of all nations.

Moreover, a number of the least developed countries have made only very limited progress: their infant, young child and maternal mortality rates and related morbidities remain unacceptably high. Projections of current trends to the year 2000 indicate that these mortality rates will persist at tragically high levels for many of those countries. For example, in many countries of Africa and Southern Asia mortality rates for children under five will still be well over 100 per thousand in the year 2000.

Health problems are also increasingly serious in large urban populations steeped in poverty.

Thus, health conditions in the least developed countries persist at levels that are so limiting and destructive of human potential and so contrary to the principles and intent of health for all, as to be unacceptable to the global community.

It is urgently necessary to recognize and acknowledge that many of the most serious health problems remain largely untouched by development efforts. These residual problems, which contribute so heavily to the human burden of death and disability, sound an insistent call for careful assessment and more vigorous application of current approaches, as well as for new approaches—new research, new mechanisms, new partnerships, new resources—in order that these problems may be overcome.

The world is faced with variable progress in pursuit of the goal of health for all, remarkable gains by many countries, modest gains by others, and, for a tragic few, little progress at all. To address the range of persisting problems and to establish preparedness for problems that will emerge in the future, the actions described below must be undertaken.

The permanence of health for all

I. Maintaining health for all as a permanent goal of all nations up to and beyond the year 2000

Reaffirm health for all as the permanent goal of all nations, as stressed in the Declaration of Alma-Ata, and establish a process for examining the longer-term challenges to health for all that will extend into the twenty-first century.

It is clear that the principles and values contained in the Declaration of Alma-Ata which underlie health for all should be seen as having a permanent place in the responsibilities of nations with respect to the health of their peoples. No nation can solve all of its health problems, and new problems continue to emerge in every country. These are biological and social realities of life.

In every nation there will be continuously changing patterns of health and disease, and always there is the national reponsibility for dealing with those problems in a way that safeguards the health of the people, ensures equity and promotes a spirit of self-reliance.

The goal of the year 2000 continues to be a milestone of great significance. Associated with it are imperatives that identified targets be met in every country, but with particular emphasis on mortality and morbidity reduction in vulnerable groups in all countries.

At the same time, it is necessary to look over the horizon, beyond the turn of the century to the problems of that time, some continuing from the present, others emerging as entirely new. The capacity for dealing with those problems needs to be strengthened further between now and the year 2000. It is likely that a very important long-term contribution of the health for all movement will be to establish in every country, and in every community, an evolving capacity to deal with the health problems of that place and time.

Thus, the goal of HFA remains unchanged, but targets will shift from those suited to the decade preceding the year 2000 to those relative to future times and places. Key principles will remain — equity, effectiveness, affordability, community participation, intersectoral collaboration. Problems will change, as will the technologies and social and organizational mechanisms to grapple with them.

Here, at the midpoint between Alma-Ata and the year 2000, the goals of all nations should be:

- to identify the critical challenges to be met between now and the turn of the century, and to make headway, even against the problems that have been most difficult to solve;
- to lay the ground for the continuing work that must follow the turn of the century, heralding appropriate changes of strategy necessary to consolidate the pursuit of health for all beyond the year 2000;
- to continue to recognize and affirm that health, peace and development are intimately related to one another, and that each must be pursued and protected, in the interests of the well-being of mankind.

Intensifying social and political action for the future—Agenda 2000

II. Renewing and strengthening strategies for health for all

Encourage each country to continue to monitor its own health problems and develop its own health strategies in the spirit of health for all. This will reveal its most pressing health problems and identify the most seriously underserved and vulnerable populations. Programmes should be directed towards those populations in a spirit of equity, inviting their active participation in the development and implementation of the strategies.

It should be acknowledged and affirmed that the concept of health for all by the year 2000, formulated at the World Health Assembly in 1977, and further elaborated at Alma-Ata in 1978, has provided the countries of the world with moral, political, social and technical guidelines that have enabled and encouraged them to deal more effectively with the problems of health inequity and ill health of their populations.

In keeping with the goal of health for all, the majority of nations and regions have made substantial progress in dealing with their problems of inequity and ineffectiveness of health services, and have significantly improved the health of their populations. All nations should continue these efforts, and, in collaboration with each other and with WHO, should pursue further targets of improvement of the health of all their people so as to ensure that every citizen has the opportunity to live a socially and economically productive life. Such improvements should go beyond physical and mental illness to the quality of life itself. Resources required to meet those targets should be identified and allocated accordingly.

In this spirit, special priority should be given to improving the health conditions of the poor and underserved, in the developed as well as the developing world, and in this way to reducing inequity. Steps should be taken to establish and pursue targets for reducing disparities in both health status and access to health services between disadvantaged population groups and the general population, for example, by reducing the differences from the national mean in under-five mortality rates, infant mortality rates and maternal mortality rates.

It has to be re-emphasized that the concept of health for all has never included the simplistic notion that the world would ever be free of health problems. The purpose of health for all is to provide a conceptual framework for thinking about the multiplicity of problems, for guiding decisions about priorities and action with a special concern for equity in health, and for sharing experiences, problems and ideas with other nations in order to promote health and reduce health inequities. It is recognized as well that both international and national policies must be adapted to local settings, where local people can bring about improvements in their own situations.

The procedures for monitoring and reporting on progress towards health for all are an important example of WHO support for sharing national experiences. They should be further strengthened to ensure that countries will benefit from each other's lessons and be inspired by examples of progress.

III. Intensifying social and political action for health

Intensify the social and political action necessary to support the shifts in policy and the allocation of resources required to progress towards health for all, including the involvement of other sectors, nongovernmental organizations, communities and other interested groups to seek mechanisms for promoting new partnerships for health among them and with governments.

Social and political action, both national and international, is imperative for progress in health development, not only to support the shifts in policy and support required to have a stronger impact on health, but also to enlist the participation of the wide variety of potentially interested parties — international organizations, nongovernmental organizations, universities, industry, student groups, individual citizens, health workers and their associations — many of whom are waiting for indications of useful directions in which to apply their resources and energies. These should be true partnerships, with active sharing of ideas, resources and responsibilities. The mass media should be used to inform others about the needs of health for all, and to advocate efforts to meet them.

Political commitment is a prerequisite to progress towards health for all, but by itself may have limited practical value. Also vital are policies which embody the commitment to work towards health for all; budgetary allocations, which are the litmus test of political commitment; structural rearrangements, which may be necessary for policy implementation; and strengthening of management, to progress towards targets and avoid excessive waste. In addition, assignment of strong leaders to key posts, and continuous support for primary health care at the district level can help to ensure that effective services reach the periphery through planned programmes rather than by only trickling down.

There is also an urgent need to challenge current international development philosophies that discount investment in health and other social sectors in favour of economic improvement only. Efforts should be undertaken to enhance the international climate for development support, including policies that focus on social equity rather than economic considerations alone, that recognize the long-term nature of social development, and that promote wider understanding and acceptance of the development process including respect for the people who are involved in its implementation. Economic policies should protect those who are most vulnerable and least able to protect themselves from economic penalties, and should recognize the contribution of social development to long-term economic progress. It is necessary to acknowledge that health is a fundamental right in addition to being a prerequisite to development.

National and international action is required to mobilize new resources, create new mechanisms and new partnerships for health development, including joint mobilization of resources between health and other sectors. WHO should assume a leadership role in this effort by promoting debate and supporting initiatives on the feasibility of new approaches in favour of the most vulnerable groups.

A special effort should be directed towards enlisting joint efforts by major developed countries towards assisting the least developed countries. Savings achieved through reductions in arms expenditure would serve this purpose well.

IV. Developing and mobilizing leadership for health for all

Give strong emphasis in every country to developing and stimulating the interest and support of current and potential leaders in the health and other sectors, at community, district and national levels, in order to bring creativity, advocacy, commitment and resources to bear on the challenge of health development.

Enlightened leadership for health for all is in short supply. Is it possible to achieve a major shift, in which those who can assume such leadership positions become more plentiful, rather than occasional, and in the front line, rather than remote from need?

At its core, health for all is a value issue. But the problems it addresses are also quantitative — all people, not some. All children are to be monitored, not some. The impact of health for all must be quantitatively effective. The numbers of people who assume leadership roles for health for all must be quantitatively significant. Their influence must be pervasive.

The quality of leadership is also vital. Those in positions where leadership is possible must understand the principles and imperatives of health for all, have a clear view of what is needed, what might be done to achieve it, how to function in their local situation to progress towards it, and how to mobilize others to join in working towards it.

There is a clear need for leadership in health and in other sectors at every level: in communities, where the need is for self-reliance; in nongovernmental organizations, where their flexibility and creativity can be brought to bear on problems of national interest; in universities, where their capacity for generating and trying new ideas and new programmes can contribute to the effectiveness of health policies and services; in government, where the responsibility resides for reaching the poorest and most deprived, and where effective policies and programmes in pursuit of health for all must be developed.

Ministries of health must deal with multiple levels of policy formulation and resource allocation, including the parliament or its equivalent. Those in policy-making roles often need support in the form of policy-related research that will assist them in formulating strategy options. Managerial leadership is required, including the capacity to manage the changes that are vital for progress towards health for all. Leadership is needed to help redress the current imbalance between social and economic development.

There is a paradox about leadership. Formally trained and experienced leaders are in short supply, and often over-used. At the same time, there are vast numbers with leadership potential who are untrained and inexperienced. Those already in leadership roles, often too few in number, need support, while at the same time opportunities for training and experience need to be created for others. Incentives need to be developed to help sustain those in leadership roles.

Beyond all else, leadership should be people-centred—people leading people in order to benefit people. The ultimate impact should be at the community level, where the need is the greatest and the opportunity to respond must be extended to those who are on the path towards self-reliance. Leadership formation must be a central theme in the larger scope of health manpower development.

V. Empowering people

Empower people by providing information, technical support and decision-making possibilities, so as to enable them to share in opportunities and responsibilities for action in the interest of their own health. Give special attention to the role of women in health and development.

Involvement of communities in primary health care is not an ethical nicety, it is a technical and social necessity. Key advances in the health of communities depend on their decisions — about how they live, care for one another and look after their environment. Important promotive, preventive, first aid and rehabilitative actions can be undertaken by people in their own homes and communities. Services that are "delivered" from outside will have limited effect unless fully understood, absorbed and taken over by communities.

Health services should fully involve communities: in defining problems, about which communities often have intimate knowledge; in decision-making, in which communities have both a right and a responsibility; in financing, where community resources can be both essential contributions and a lever to ensure that the people's voice is heeded. Health services need to reach the home, family and place of work, through local people trained in or near the community, to provide ready access to health assistance as required. Health personnel must learn how to organize and support community involvement.

The role of women in promoting healthy ways of life is essential. They need to be given opportunities for self-improvement and to contribute to the development and quality of life in their communities, including extending their activities beyond family life to policy-making and implementation. Education alone may not suffice to put women in positions to take effective action — some degree of autonomy or independence is required for them to make decisions and take actions necessary to promote improvements in health for themselves and their families. Empowering women includes giving them control over their own lives, bodies and family size.

Health is mainly determined in the home and the workplace, where families live and work in healthy or unhealthy ways, where behaviour is influenced by family, neighbours and fellow workers, and where decisions are made that affect every aspect of family health. People must be given information about their health and how it can be improved. For them to lack such knowledge leads to both dependence and ignorance, neither of which has a place in community development. People should participate in determining what kinds of information and education they need for their individual community development. The views of health professionals about community needs may conflict with people's perceptions — differences that require harmonization through better dialogue. Health services must help people to learn how to care for themselves.

The health of the family depends on the health status of all family members; the father and other members of the household should not be overlooked, even though priority is given to the mother and children. Attention to the others, through assessment of their health risks, also serves the interests of the mother and children, and supports the integrity of the family unit. Empowerment should go beyond mothers and fathers to their children, tomorrow's generation, who can be reached through schools and youth groups.

VI. Making intersectoral collaboration a force for health for all

Support the creation of sustained intersectoral collaboration for health by incorporating health objectives into the public policies of other sectors and activating potential mechanisms at all levels.

It is widely recognized that health is not the concern of the health sector alone but is dependent on the actions of many social and economic sectors, both governmental and nongovernmental. Education for literacy, income supplementation, clean water and adequate sanitation, improved housing, ecological sustainability, food and other agricultural products, building of roads — all may have a substantial and synergistic impact on health. However, few innovative examples exist of sustained intersectoral collaboration for health.

It is apparent that sectoral priorities and administrative structures usually preclude the sharing of ideas, joint planning and collaborative action. This problem has been exacerbated by poor advocacy and lack of commitment to the idea of intersectoral collaboration by the health sector itself.

At the very time when lack of resources for health is universally proclaimed as a most serious problem, it is neither rational nor defensible to ignore the potential of shared responsibility between sectors. Intersectoral collaboration must be made a force for achieving health for all.

Many practical possibilities for action exist. Identification of vulnerable groups and cross-sectoral assessment of their needs can provide the basis for collaboration at community level. Involvement in the process by people themselves adds to its effectiveness. Existing intersectoral mechanisms such as district development committees need to be further utilized by the health sector. This will require more effective advocacy on the part of health personnel in relating to other sectors. At national level, ways of strengthening sectoral policies need to be found so as to maximize the impact of health-enhancing actions while eliminating or reducing the impact of those that are harmful. The particular energies and interests of nongovernmental organizations may serve as important catalysts in all of these.

At all levels research jointly pursued by collaborating sectors can be an important tool for identifying ways of making intersectoral collaboration work.

Accelerating action for health for all — Agenda 2000

VII. Strengthening district health systems based on primary health care

Strengthen district health systems based on primary health care, as a key action point for focusing national policies and resources and local concerns on the most pressing health needs and on underserved people.

District health systems based on primary health care should be at the centre of the health for all effort. Acceptance of primary health care is fairly general at policy levels, but implementation that achieves widespread coverage is often absent, especially in the least developed countries. The problem is only partly due to scarcity of resources. There are weaknesses in planning, management, financing and evaluation capacities, and in training and providing effective support for personnel in field settings.

More attention needs to be given to strengthening health infrastructures. Given an effective infrastructure, primary health care programmes can be added or deleted according to local need, targeted at specific problems. Emphasis should be on integrated or comprehensive primary health care, in contrast to selective or vertical structures, which often lead to overconcentration of limited resources on a few programmes, and disruption of efforts to strengthen health systems based on primary health care as an integral part of community development.

A further deficiency is the inability and even disinterest in monitoring simple indicators of coverage and health status. These deficiencies result in systems that are blind to programme results and powerless to correct drift or failure. Here is the key to the heart of the health for all challenge — equity. Without a system design that can achieve coverage, without simple indicators to identify inequities and measure success or failure in dealing with them, without effective management, including a capacity for self-correction, without involving the community at all levels, equity becomes a lost hope.

Another weakness is the lack of supportive interaction between the district and higher levels of health services on the one hand, and with community level activities on the other. Strongly centralized decision-making discourages initiative at the periphery, while exclusive interest in health facilities and doctor-based services results in little support to community level activities. TCDV — Technical Cooperation among Developing Villages — can be encouraged through district health systems. To facilitate such activities, decentralization to district and community levels is essential.

The district is well suited to overcoming problems of health services in relation to community development including: preparation of health personnel for effective functioning in district programmes; management technologies; interaction with communities; and intersectoral working relationships.

Vital interactions between the primary-, secondary- and tertiary-care levels of a health system are usually missing in health services, and the district health system is the ideal place to develop them. One of the most difficult linkages to establish among the levels of health services is between the front-line or district hospital and community-based primary health care. Maternity services, based in the community and backed up by the front-line hospital, are one example of a challenge to primary health care that demands effective linkages in order to save the lives of women with complications of pregnancy and delivery.

VIII. Planning, preparing and supporting health personnel for health for all

Reorient education and training programmes for health personnel, emphasizing relevance to health services requirements, by locating learning experiences in functioning health systems based on primary health care. Provide strong moral and resource support for personnel, particularly those working in remote areas or difficult circumstances.

The deficiencies are deep and widespread — professionals inadequately trained or motivated to work where the needs are. Three aspects of health manpower development need emphasis:

- Recruitment and training are too often separated entirely from planning and utilization—a reason for WHO's emphasis on integrated health systems and manpower development (HSMD). But the integration must be more than a paper exercise; education and training should relate to and also take place in field settings where operational primary health care programmes embody a large part of the desired manpower competencies. Training and uses of community and auxiliary level personnel need to be closely related to those of other health workers. Health manpower policies should be consistent with national health for all strategies.

- The preparation of health personnel needs to be strengthened in terms of relevance to health services and to people's health needs and demands, as in competency-based, community-oriented, team-focused learning experiences, and also in terms of educational methodologies, as in community-based, problem-oriented, student-oriented, self-learning experiences. More than academic jargon, these are key ideas in the interactions between education and function.

- Less well appreciated is the severe demoralization of health personnel in many field settings, particularly in more remote locations. The neglect and unresponsiveness of health services in this respect are consistent, widespread and destructive. Neglect often leads to a sense of uselessness and lack of motivation, and, when such despondency occurs, loss of dependability and integrity is not far behind. Better management practices and personnel support systems could incorporate supportive policies, such as: incentives for exemplary work and assignment in hardship settings; amenities to improve the quality of family life; continuing education; and career development opportunities.

Universities and other training institutions have key roles to play in addressing these issues, by linking their educational, research and services programmes directly with national plans for health system and manpower development. Universities should be involved in community-based primary health care activities where various kinds of students can learn, as team members, how to address health and health system problems in community settings. Early exposure to community-based problems, and to interactions of epidemiology and management can be emphasized. In these settings, students can also learn about the needs of field-based health personnel for support and professional encouragement.

Thus, the concept of health system and manpower development leads the university beyond the more traditional concept of the teaching hospital to a teaching health system. Through association with a functioning health system, the university has the opportunity for ensuring close relevance between educational preparation and national needs, and also for contributing to improvements in the field-based health services research.

IX. Ensuring the development and rational use of science and appropriate technology

Emphasize the applications of science and appropriate technology to the critical health problems that threaten populations in all parts of the world, and strengthen the research capacities of Third World countries, with emphasis on research aimed at improving the health of the most deprived people.

Science has much to offer health for all. Some problems call for advanced scientific insight and methodologies almost on an emergency scale, as in grappling with the AIDS pandemic. There are other calls on science, some less dramatic, but no less important, for example new applications of diagnostic methods that can be used in remote locations. New vaccines will strengthen health services, and new techniques for the control of tropical diseases will ease the burden of suffering on countless lives.

However, the most serious deficiencies in improving health in developing countries do not relate to a shortage of technology, but to inadequacies of health system infrastructures and the high cost of making technology available to all in need. This fundamental deficiency is often compounded by the indiscriminate transfer of technology to developing countries. The result is the consumption of scarce resources which would be used more effectively in primary health care programmes.

Assessment of the costs and impacts of alternative technologies has an important place. The costs of the transfer of technology may be more than that of the technology itself. Application of existing knowledge and technology — when they are effective — is an essential first step. The utility of traditional versus modern technologies needs to be kept in view. Good maintenance can reduce overall costs and ensure reliable functioning of equipment. Educational methods are an important consideration in transferring appropriate technology from country to country and sector to sector.

Most health problems of developing countries cannot be solved by indiscriminate technology transfer. Solutions must be developed on the spot, and capacity-building in research is essential, based on a clear view of the range of technological choices involved, and a detailed knowledge of local research capacities. This is an ideal enterprise for North-South collaboration. Emerging needs for enhanced research capacity must be addressed in the context of extreme resource constraints and the search begun, none the less, for new resources, new mechanisms, and new partners. Operations research and health services research have great practical usefulness in dealing with problems at field level.

Attention should also be given to the ethical implications of advances in technology. When the technology is beneficial but costly, questions of equity and autonomy arise: who should benefit and who should be passed by, and what are the roles of individuals and communities in making such decisions?

Thus, a balanced strategy is needed for applying the benefits of science and technology to health worldwide. There should be strong support for the enhancement of scientific research and education in all countries. Continued global efforts should be directed towards strengthening health research capacities of scientists from developing countries and their institutions, so they might collaborate in a global research network.

X. Overcoming problems that continue to resist solution

Establish priority programmes aimed at overcoming serious problems, where underdevelopment or disturbances in development are major contributing factors and progress has been very limited, such as high infant, child and maternal mortality rates, abuse of substances such as tobacco and alcohol, and the imbalance between population growth and environmental and socioeconomic resources. Develop improved approaches through primary health care, emphasizing intersectoral action.

The most serious problems to be addressed between now and the year 2000 will be those that resist solution largely because of underlying conditions of severe underdevelopment, as in the least developed countries, or long-established patterns of personal and social behaviour, as in developed countries. It is necessary to be clear, however, that the people are not the causes of these problems, they are the victims — of underdevelopment or "development-gone-wrong" — and solutions must address those development problems at their roots, and not simply blame people for circumstances the world has given them. Examples can be taken from both developed and developing countries:

Very high maternal and under-five mortality rates. Sixty-four countries with 40% of the world's population suffer more than 80% of the under-five deaths, and more than 90% of maternal deaths occurring in the world each year. These high death rates are embedded in the problems of underdevelopment — poverty, malnutrition, illiteracy, and contaminated environments — and remain unresolved in a large number of countries despite widespread knowledge of how to deal with the problems.

Underdevelopment, population growth and environment. A number of developing countries face serious problems of socioeconomic underdevelopment: ineffective agricultural development, landlessness of populations, migration of rural populations to urban centres, poverty, weakness of health systems, including family planning services based on primary health care, and poor environmental health. These examples show the importance of a multisectoral approach to the solution of health problems on the part of national authorities and international organizations.

The expanding use of tobacco and its commercial exploitation. The continued use of tobacco in developed countries, and its expanding use in developing countries, with commercialization pursued in the face of irrefutable scientific evidence of human harm is an example of a global problem that calls for continued aggressive action to combat it at all levels: political, social, scientific and economic.

Other examples can be given of problems embedded in the process of development in both developing and developed countries: alcohol and drug abuse; environmental pollution; an enlarging and dependent population of elderly people; unwanted pregnancies and illegal abortions.

Efforts to address these problems must be directed at the underlying problems of development. Primary health care, with its strong emphasis on intersectoral collaboration provides avenues for addressing the problems. However, new approaches are also called for: new ways of analysing the problems, new approaches to field-based research, new forms of interacting with other sectors, and new scales of action.

Special priority initiative in support of the least developed countries by WHO and the international community

> **Establish a special international initiative focused on the tragic circumstances of the least developed countries, mostly on the continent of Africa, and especially those with markedly elevated infant, under-five-year-old and maternal mortality rates, which will address specific obstacles to progress and will set targets to be reached by the year 2000.**

While most countries have benefited from the health for all movement, a tragic residue is suffering from death and disability, so extreme as to leave no doubt that they are being by-passed by even the barest of opportunities to progress towards a minimal level of human dignity and well-being.

It must be appreciated that these nations are not the cause of their problems of development stagnation; rather they are the victims of it. They have been marginalized by it, and to a large extent they have been abandoned to it. The resources and processes involved in international development have failed these people, and the health for all effort has thus far failed them as well.

In order to confront this unacceptable situation it is proposed that the World Health Assembly declare its commitment to helping these tragedy-ridden countries fully into the development process. This will require special and urgent priority on the part of WHO to support the poorest countries, particularly those with the highest infant, under-five, and maternal mortality rates. More extensive resources and stronger commitment than hitherto available are urgently needed.

The World Health Assembly should further undertake to monitor the outcome of this effort. The rate of progress should serve as an indicator of the effectiveness of the resolve of Member States in dealing with this most fundamental of challenges — countries that, without effective development assistance and collaboration, will probably slip further down the spiral of development failure.

Forty-first
World Health Assembly

The significance of the Forty-first World Health Assembly

The World Health Assembly is the supreme authority of the World Health Organization. This annual meeting brings together hundreds of people — national delegations, representatives of international organizations and nongovernmental organizations, and the staff of WHO, some from the head-quarters in Geneva, many others from the six regions of the Organization.

The World Health Assembly is a remarkable aggregation of people. National delegations, many with high levels of technical expertise, arrive with critical experiences in their home settings and often with diplomatic instructions regarding positions to take on items on the Assembly's agenda. Representatives of international organizations come with the intention of strengthening col-laboration with WHO and with its Member countries. From nongovernmental organizations come individuals seeking better understanding of the problems of world health and the programmes of WHO, so that they can make their own programmes more relevant and effective; and conversely to enlighten WHO as to the potential of nongovernmental organizations. The staff of WHO is alert to reactions of delegations to programmes that WHO has implemented, and look for indications of new directions that countries and agencies might want to take.

The debates in the main committees and plenary sessions, the conversations in the corridors and coffee shop, the notes exchanged, the nods of acknowledge-ment or understanding — these form complex interactions that are the essence of communication at the World Health Assembly.

From this rich and complex mix of people, ideas, and professional collabora-tion emerge the critical initiatives and decisions of the Assembly that shape the strategies and programmes of WHO.

It was in this milieu that the decision was made in 1975 to proceed with an international conference that was to take place at Alma-Ata. It was in 1980 that the strategy for health for all found its final form, built on recommenda-tions from the six regions of the world. It was here, year after year, in the decade since Alma-Ata that the hopes and scepticism, the initiatives and evalua-tions, the informal discussions and formal proposals, as well as planning for shifts in strategy to strengthen health for all took place.

It was here, in May 1988, that a new convergence took place, this time reviving historical material from Alma-Ata, distributing ideas that had emerged from Riga, describing experiences and voicing opinions about what had happened since Alma-Ata. There was a drawing together of all of this into reflections by the Director-General, the debate on leadership for health for all in the Technical Discussions, thoughtful remarks by round table experts, and, finally, the adoption of a resolution on strengthening primary health care. Here the threads of historical experience, insight, hope and determination have been somehow pulled together into the current understanding of Alma-Ata — what started there, what has happened since, and what the prospects are for the future.

At the World Health Assembly there were several distinct events that were to have a direct bearing on the theme of Alma-Ata:

- The Director-General's report[1] to the Health Assembly, examining the status of world health and the forces that bear on it, as he saw them. He referred extensively to universal principles for health, many of which found their origins in the spirit of Alma-Ata.

- The Director-General's remarks[2] on the fortieth anniversary of WHO. The celebration of 40 years since the founding of the Organization included remarks by delegates representing six regions and also by the Director-General.

- The Technical Discussions on the subject of Leadership Development for Health for All,[3] the product of several years of careful planning and programmatic action by the WHO staff and Member nations.

- The round table debate on the tenth anniversary of Alma-Ata.[4] Here was the high point of the Assembly with respect to reflections on Alma-Ata. A dozen experts, from all parts of the world, many of whom were at Alma-Ata, reflected on the theme of Alma-Ata's continuing contribution to world health.

- The Health Assembly's resolution[5] designed to contribute to the further strengthening of primary health care. This key resolution accepted the reaffirmation of Alma-Ata from Riga and incorporated the action steps recommended there as well as on the floor of the Assembly.

---

[1] See page 91.
[2] See page 98.
[3] See page 104.
[4] See page 110.
[5] See page 152.

World health — 2000 and beyond

Address by Dr H. Mahler, Director-General, to the World Health Assembly, 3 May 1988

Mr President, honourable delegates, ladies and gentlemen, *ce n'est pas des lois qu'il faut parler, c'est des moeurs.* It is not of laws that we should speak, it is of morals. The French social philosopher, Montesquieu, expressed sentiments to that effect nearly 250 years ago. They are as pertinent today as they were then. The quest for morality in human affairs laid the spiritual foundation then, and in subsequent centuries, for social revolutions aimed at political equity. It has laid the spiritual foundation today for another kind of social revolution aimed at health equity. **For without vision inspired by morality, the goal of health for all by the year 2000 could never have been conceived. And without that same vision and that same morality it will never be attained.**

Its attainment depends on health systems based on primary health care, the theme of your general debate this year. These are highly practical matters. But there are different kinds of practicality. One is the kind that is all too rampant in our present-day, largely amoral, world. I am referring to short-sighted, spiritless pragmatism devoid of vision. But there is another kind—pragmatism infused with morality. It is on that kind that I should like to dwell today.

The concept of "health" and the meaning of "all" have to be taken together to understand properly the significance of "health for all". In order to understand that, and to appreciate the means for attaining it, it is useful to compare the concept and the means with those of the past.

Perhaps the greatest difference between the health concepts and practices of yester-year and those of recent decades has been their concentration, in the past, on individuals and, at present, on society as a whole — from the smallest village to the entire world.

In the distant past, the art of health lay in healing individuals, even if that included wise advice on personal habits. The healers understood the importance of the environment — water and air in particular — but they did not know how to control it, and some even adopted fatalistic attitudes. In spite of differences of viewpoints, Hippocrates and Aesculapius shared that concern for individuals turning to them for help. The daughters of Aesculapius — Hygeia the goddess of health and Panacea the divine healer of all ailments — were siblings but not twins, and Panacea, the healer, was the favourite.

The individual as a patient continued to be the focus of medieval masters of medicine. And when some traditional systems of medicine tried to cope with the health problems of their local community, they did so in much the same way as they tried to exorcise the evil spirits of disease from individuals. It was only in the course of the past century that a handful of social policy-makers with vision grasped that ensuring the wholesomeness of water and air and housing and workplaces was crucial for the health of communities. But the vision was limited mainly to those surrounding them. When they considered the health of distant communities they tended to divide them into two camps — those they considered to be of similar social standing and therefore to have similar interests of self-protection, and the others to be protected against. The first attempts at international health, lasting for a century, provide ample evidence of the aim of protecting the North from the infiltration of the health problems of the South. From our perspective, that was a very far cry from international morality. But then our perspective has changed radically over the past half century.

I shall explain. It has become commonplace to state that science and technology in general, and health science and technology in particular, have made greater strides over the past few decades than throughout the whole of the rest of human history. What is perhaps less apparent, but no less startling, is that health policy in general, and international health policy in particular, have made greater strides over the past few decades than throughout the whole of preceding human history. Just as the twentieth century has seen the evolution of universal principles to explain the physical world, and later the biological world, recent years have seen the emergence of principles governing health throughout the world.

These principles take into account that, if people have changed little genetically over the course of known history, throughout large parts of the world they have radically changed the environment surrounding them. Sound social policy for health is, therefore, more important than ever, to ensure a correct balance between the biological make-up of people and the physical and social environment in which they live — that balance which is of the very essence of health. Under the influence of technological euphoria, it is so easy to become blind and deaf to the differing needs of people living under different socioeconomic and cultural circumstances, particularly when communication technology transmits information at electromagnetic speed, mainly in one direction. Unfortunately, international developmental efforts over the past few decades have fallen into that trap.

Going back thirty-odd years, to the 1950s — and I have a personal experience of what I am going to say because I spent those years in my second mother country, India — going back to those years, the bilateral and multilateral agencies behaved as though colonialism was going to last for ever, except that they were going to take over from the erstwhile colonizing powers. These agencies behaved towards the countries on which they were inflicting technical assistance in a very paternalistic, supranational way. They had not learned that you cannot bring about social and economic development by proxy. The tragedy is that neither had the countries receiving the assistance realized that. They regarded their apparent benefactors as beggars do, not realizing that charity enslaves — both those who receive and those who give — because it leaves little or nothing behind beyond survival in misery.

Then came the 1960s, the euphoria created by the emergence of politically independent states from former colonies and an over-optimistic aura of economic boom. Large-scale was the order of the day — large-scale parodies of development in the form of exported economic growth projects. Yes, I call them parodies, although there was nothing funny about them, because they had little in common with what development initiative *should* be all about — and that is to start from the axiom that people *do* matter, and therefore to reinforce people's energy as the most important input into social and economic productivity. Instead, the entire focus was on economic growth, with no sensitivity whatsoever to the concept of social poverty, and to the need to support people in extricating themselves from that.

Even when the need was realized to coordinate international assistance, rather than squandering resources in widely differing directions, even then the international community believed it could achieve results by planning together through some sort of second and third guessing in the capital cities of the industrialized world, far far away from the theatre of operations. The futility had still not been grasped of attempting development as though the people in the developing countries did not exist but only the material world did. Little or no attempt was made to develop the capacities of the people of these countries to define their social and economic development needs.

The climate seemed to begin to change in the 1970s. I say "seemed" because fundamentally little changed. True, many governments in both developing and developed countries began to give greater thought to social policy, as individuals and groups of people of all ideological shades were doing. Such notions as "social relevance" and "social justice" became current language. The environment became a subject of wide international concern. But by the end of the 1970s, developmental inertia, inability to shake off old dogmas, a worsening economic situation in many countries, particularly the developing ones, and total preoccupation with solely material values and political action for material gain all led to severe disillusionment over human development and any kind of external intervention that could possibly promote it.

So, in the 1980s, the international community had reached a stage of developmental crisis, ready only for crisis management. Too many countries, too many bilateral and multilateral agencies, too many influential individuals had become too disillusioned with the prospects for genuine human development to be ready to continue the struggle for it. No wonder they clutched at the straw of emergency aid. Even that great Swedish developmental humanist whom I so revere — Gunnar Myrdal — even he reached the conclusion that the only useful form of international support to the developing countries was emergency aid.

Honourable delegates, what bearing, you might ask, do these philosophical meanderings have on the attainment of health for all through health systems based on primary health care? Well, in spite of the developmental dialogue of the deaf I have just outlined — in spite of that — and in spite of political and ideological strife in so many parts of the world, in an amazingly short time by any standards collective health policies were defined that sowed the seeds of social revolution in community health. If I have bewailed the absence of real dialogue between North and South in relation to development in

93

general, fortunately this dialogue — East and West and North and South — has taken place with respect to health. It has led to the definition of the universal principles for health that I mentioned a few moments ago. It has also led to action for health based on these principles. That action still has to be greatly intensified. It is therefore timely to recapitulate the principles on which it should be based.

The first principle is to define social policies for health that are relevant not only for individuals but for societies as a whole, and to apply universal physical and biological principles in morally sound ways, leading to greater equity and decency in health matters and empathy for the underprivileged. The vision of health for all by the year 2000 was inspired by such a sense of morality. It echoed Gunnar Myrdal's dying words: "We must not let the injustices of the world take over". The vision came as a conscience-stricken response to the indecency of so much preventable ill health throughout the world and of the growing gap between the health "haves" and the health "have nots". This gap was striking and remains striking, within countries and among countries. The vision came at a time when it had become increasingly clear that the health of individuals and of the society in which they live are closely interconnected.

To improve the health of any society, it is necessary to raise the level of health of its less privileged members. That is not only an epidemiological truism, it is a moral obligation. It is the principle of principles that has crystallized out since WHO was born.

Health for all was conceived initially for the underprivileged, but it has been used much more profitably by the privileged. The industrialized countries therefore owe a social debt to the developing ones, if only on that score alone, and who knows to what extent that debt counterbalances the financial debts in the opposite direction! Surely that is additional reason for the moral conscience of all of us to continue to trouble us and to incite us to repay that social debt, by keeping the needs of the developing countries first and foremost in our minds, and by supporting them in ways that *they* require.

This brings me to one of the universal principles for health that is enshrined in the Declaration of Alma-Ata, and that is the self-reliance of individuals, communities and whole countries. If it is moral to be charitable for short periods in order to tide people and countries over difficult times, I do not consider it moral to subjugate them to long-standing dependency. That only destroys their personality and corrupts the self-styled donors. Investments have to be made to help people to understand what makes or breaks health and how they can shape their own health as well as the health of their families and the community in which they live. So here is another universal principle — people *can* be important social carriers of their own health destiny. And yet another principle — the moral imperative of ensuring that people have access to objective, valid information on all aspects of health that concern them — information that is presented in ways that make it semantically and culturally understandable by them so that they can comprehend it and act on it.

Being properly informed not only contributes to people's capacity to cope with their health, it is an important factor in their social productivity. The meaning of social productivity in the goal of health for all has been much too neglected. It is a powerful indicator *of* health and a powerful lever *for* health. It implies the contribution that people can make to the social development of the community in which they live. They can make that contribution in many forums — within the family, among their friends and acquaintances, at their places of work or of learning, in social groups and in nongovernmental organizations. And they can do so in a wide variety of ways, such as social support, voluntary action for the health of society, literature, art, music, sport, cultural practice and the shaping of public policies. These are the ways by which people build vibrant societies and are themselves built in the course of doing so. That kind of productivity makes all the difference between apathetic societies, devoid of communal souls, and dynamic societies full of the vigour of life. That dynamism is essential for economic development. So here is another universal principle that transcends the boundaries of health: social productivity is essential for economic productivity. Those countries that have not realized that, and have done little to foster the social productivity of their people, have done so at the peril of economic stagnation, and have mortgaged their future development.

Here then is yet another universal principle that has come to light in recent decades: health and socioeconomic development go hand in hand in mutually reinforcing ways. The application of the recently discovered principles for health can in itself be a useful option for achieving socioeconomic progress, as many developing countries in particular have been fortunate enough to learn, and sufficiently satisfied to state in public. That principle has been repeated many times in this forum. It has now penetrated such financial sanctuaries as the World Bank and the International Monetary Fund, as well as a string of developmental agencies. But it cannot be repeated often enough. The message must reverberate in other forums too.

For when morality and economics join forces, that is surely a solid basis for optimism about the social and economic future of humanity. It is not just economic *adjustment* with a human face that we need to foster; it is economic *development* with a human face.

Nobody expects economic development to happen by inertia; it requires acts of volition. So does health development. Another recently discovered principle is that it is possible to set targets for health, and to attain them. Smallpox eradication was a striking example of this. Another striking example is child immunization. By setting a target, and striving to attain it, coverage has risen from 5% to more than 50% of the world's children within a decade. To succeed it is necessary to be proactive, not merely reactive. It is necessary to apply good management, and that includes open-minded research and development and the use of relevant, sensitive and consistent information. The management of health systems is appalling in far too many countries, but at least we have learned of its importance and have at our disposal relatively straightforward universal principles for good management. We have also learned to distinguish between management and bureaucracy. Good management based on

95

democratic involvement of the different levels of the health system releases human potential; bad bureaucracy, concentrating all decision-making power in central authority, stifles human potential and social productivity.

We also have at our disposal a vast array of technology for preventing disease, diagnosing it, curing it, and caring for and rehabilitating those in need. In our quest for health for all we have come to realize that these are not separate entities. We have come to understand that Hygeia, the preventer, and Panacea, the healer, are not only sisters, they are twin sisters, difficult to dissociate from each other. In this complex of health care, technology abounds — a triumph for research, a tribute to human ingenuity, and often a blessing if properly used. Yet this is a field in which morality must abound too; no amount of artificial intelligence in machines can substitute for morality in people — selling, or donating or using these machines. How often is morality conspicuous by its absence in these areas! How often do we find derelict buildings and equipment in developing countries, sold or donated without thought for their social relevance or for the economic capacity of the country to use them! Worse, how often are countries subjugated technically and crippled financially by having inappropriate technology foisted on them by others, in what amounts to an enforced return to the worship of idols in the form of shiny devices! Fortunately, we now have at our disposal universal principles for assessing the appropriateness of health technology. Not only must that technology be scientifically sound; it must be socially acceptable, both to those on whom it is used and to those who use it, and it must be economically affordable by the country concerned. In addition, social and behavioural measures may be no less important than technical ones. It *is* possible to assess the appropriateness of health technology in these terms, and that can make all the difference between the rational use of health technology — rationality being the life blood of science — and its irrational use, in spite of scientific research having conceived it.

We have become aware in recent years of the possibility of promoting health as distinct from preventing disease. Some measures to that end can be taken by the health sectors; others lie more in the domain of other sectors — education, environment, agriculture, industry, communications and the like. So we have another important universal principle. Health is a social and political aspiration that depends heavily on commitment to it at the highest levels of government, and on the coordinated action of a number of sectors. It also depends on action by communities in which the separateness of sectors becomes an artificial constraint.

Once it was realized that health systems have to be proactive rather than reactive, that health can be planned for, that it can be targeted for, and that specific programmes can be designed to attain the targets, once that was realized, the organization of health systems and all the human and other resources needed to set them up and manage them became more important than ever. This led to the principle of the health system infrastructure, that aggregate of services, organizations, institutions, and those operating them, to deliver a variety of health programmes. And it led to the understanding that all of these components have to be well planned, well organized, well coordinated and well administered. This is radically different from previous practice of waiting for people to turn up as patients before taking action.

To set up health systems that are based on the principles I have referred to requires a rare blend of vision and pragmatism. Vision without pragmatism is like an ethereal soul. Pragmatism without vision is like a shapeless body. Pragmatism within vision adds body to soul. To attain such a combination needs leadership.

That is another principle we have learned. To steer the movement of health for all towards the year 2000 and beyond requires dedicated leadership. That leadership is required not only at central levels of government; it is needed at all levels of organized society, and in all walks of life. To provide that leadership, people are required whose ennobling ideas, and words, and personal example fire the imagination of others and give rise to inspired action. Health systems based on socially indifferent pragmatism can be managed by robots. Health systems based on the principles I have been recalling can only be managed by people imbued with moral principles. So once more the importance of moral integrity becomes abundantly apparent. But that is not enough; leaders have to lead in the right direction and use the right means, and to do that requires the right balance between emotional energy and logical thinking. That may seem to be asking for too much, but even the limited experience of the past few years has demonstrated that health leaders *can* be cultivated, and *must* be cultivated, if the movement towards health for all is to increase in momentum.

At the international level, that leadership has been provided by your WHO, made possible by the high moral standing that has become its hallmark. If universal principles for health are there to guide us, most of the credit must go to your Organization. That morally responsible leadership must continue, not for the glory of WHO but for the benefit of people everywhere. So much depends on you, the World Health Assembly, collectively ensuring its continuity. Much depends, too, on your individual steadfastness in applying the principles for health that your Organization has placed at the disposal of the world.

If you maintain your faith in human development and in the important contribution of health to that development; if you act as the international social carriers of health; if you do everything in your power to mobilize the human and financial resources required to improve the health of people everywhere; if you apply in your countries the universal principles for health that have been defined in your WHO; if you insist on your governments following these principles as part of their developmental efforts; if you impart these principles to your people and inspire them to use them in their struggle to improve their own health and the health of the society in which they live; if you use these principles in your bilateral and multilateral relationships, in a spirit of equal rights to health of the people living in the South, North, East and West of spaceship earth; if you insist on *your* Organization, *your* WHO, continuing to lead the way to better health throughout the world through action guided by the vision that inspired these principles and that could inspire further beneficial innovations in the future; if you do all of that, you will lead the world and all its people to ever better health and ever greater social justice.

Mr President, honourable delegates, some of you have helped to shape these universal principles for health. Others of you have inherited them from your predecessors. All of us are morally obligated to hand them on to our successors. That is the way of life. Generations come and generations go, but what distinguishes human beings from all other animals is our ability to transfer our legacy of knowledge and culture from one generation to another.

Our universal principles for health are a precious legacy. They are a living legacy that has to be acted out and refined as new problems arise and new solutions are found. That legacy has to be continually transferred, inside countries, among countries, worldwide. And it has to be transferred inside your Organization and outside it. You are its guardians. Guard it carefully! Use it wisely! For it is the key that will open the doors of health towards the year 2000 and far beyond, well into the third millenium.

So let me conclude by paraphrasing one of my favourite statements by George Bernard Shaw "The problems of our world cannot be solved by sceptics or cynics, whose horizons are limited by obvious realities. We need women and men who can dream of things that never were and ask: Why not?" Health for all — why not?

Remarks by Dr H. Mahler, Director-General, to the World Health Assembly on the Fortieth Anniversary of WHO, 4 May 1988

I am very often asked what have been WHO's greatest achievements throughout the 40 years of its existence. Of course I could answer by giving smart, shining examples of great programme successes, and I always have this temptation, as you indeed have, to start with the super victory of eradicating smallpox from spaceship earth, not only because of its intrinsic humane value but because all of you, because of that single victory, have got all your contributions to WHO in all its 40 years back with interest. What are we talking about, when you cannot pay your contribution to WHO? One single truth. Of course with my vanity complex I could also speak about tuberculosis and the transfer of technology from one developing country to the industrialized countries, helping them to introduce ambulatory care and closing down the sanitoria, saving them billions of dollars, because of WHO's ability to reach the scientific consensus on ambulatory treatment as something totally acceptable and equally efficacious as hospital treatment. Then I could add with a little kind of pleasure that tuberculosis is now actually declining in most developing countries too, because that is what gives a little kick to my heart.

Of course I could add many more success stories that have been initiated by your WHO. Who would have thought this among you the cynics and sceptics? When you, the World Health Assembly, said we should be immunizing all the world's children by 1990 against the major killers of childhood desease,

I do not think anybody believed we could get anywhere; and I am not saying we are there altogether, but at least we have moved from less than 5% ten years ago to more than 50% fully immunized children in the world, saving more — and way more — than a million children from dying from these diseases, or becoming crippled by poliomyelitis. And if you look at the diarrhoeal disease programme, we now also have results there, saving more than one million children from dying from diarrhoea. Indeed, I would like to challenge you. On the basis of these results, what about having the guts to suggest that we should eradicate poliomyelitis from spaceship earth by the year 2000? I think we should, I think it is "do-able" and therefore there is not any excuse for not trying, and trying very hard, to do it. Other landmarks are many — for instance, not only the introduction of the concept of essential drugs but putting it to practical use, which is changing the health care scene in many developing countries today. If you look at field trials or break-through drugs for a large number of devastating parasitic diseases — I need only mention mefloquin, ivermectin, praziquantel and the like — you will see that your WHO has been in business. I could mention to you our trials now for new vaccines against leprosy, typhoid and cholera, the strategy for preventing coronary heart diseases and lung cancer, and making available to the world a low-cost, highly effective basic system for diagnostic radiology. And of course I could also among these spectaculars, end up by saying to you: do you think anybody else could have done what we have been doing about AIDS in less than one year or in a year's time, putting that into motion, so that we have gained credibility everywhere in the world? I do not think so.

I have given here a menu of only a very few examples of WHO's successes. But I would not dwell on these, not because I do not think they are important — I think they are highly important. But there are also other products of your WHO, which normally are a little bit forgotten.

I think your Organization has brought about a fundamental change in our very understanding of health and ways of attaining it. It has made a unique contribution to the restoration of social justice. It has demonstrated that health can be achieved by all and not just by the privileged few. It has shown how health goals can be arrived at out of ethical values in a highly materialistic world. It has displayed empathy for people in a highly egoistical world and sincerity in a most cynical world. It has transferred technology transparently and honestly in a technically mystified world. And it has done all that rationally, although not unemotionally, in a highly irrational world.

I suppose the most outstanding way in which your Organization is displaying these qualities is in its Strategy, so-called "Health for all by the year 2000", and of course maintaining that goal long beyond the year 2000. I always repeat that this Strategy is outstanding for the values it represents. It was born out of desperation at the appalling health of underprivileged people, particularly in the developing countries. And you know that desperation so easily leads to nihilism. Instead, thanks to the climate in your Organization, it led to a very constructive positivism. That attitude, coupled with the knowledge that sufficient technology does exist that could easily be afforded by countries throughout the world, if they were willing to set their priorities right, that attitude and that knowledge led WHO to come forward, you to come forward in the face of conventional wisdom, in the face of cynics and sceptics, with this dramatic social challenge for the end of the twentieth century.

But your Organization did not content itself by being just the world's health conscience; it acted in response to that conscience and it acted very swiftly. Just ten years ago, shortly after the health-for-all enunciation, WHO with its favourite consort, UNICEF, went together with you and so many other nongovernmental organizations to Alma-Ata and issued the Declaration of Alma-Ata, which by any reckoning is a historic manifesto. It enshrines indeed a new paradigm for health and provides a way of converting health for all into practicalities through health systems based on primary health care.

For the first time, thanks to you, your WHO, the world has a set of universal principles for health, a social helix whose strands can shape many different health systems in response to different needs and different capacities.

In this way your Organization has, like it or not, given rise to new hope in developing countries and a new interest in health in industrialized countries. In many developing countries the strands are being put together in such a way as to offer a totally new approach to social and economic development; and in many industrialized countries they are being put together to attain defined targets for improved health through better deployment of existing resources. And your Organization has shown how the economically privileged countries can really support the less privileged ones through the enlightened application of the principles, the collective principles for health that you, through your WHO, have placed at the disposal of all countries.

Sure, we do not know everything. You have, in this Assembly, tried to put forward the idea of the district health system; but we still have a very long way to go before we really grasp the managerial intricacies of making good district programmes. And therefore I would like to make a parting appeal to you that I consider it almost scandalous how little WHO has invested in research and development to try to support countries to find out how you can really get optimal managerial approaches to delivering your meagre resources. I think it is high time to redress this very considerable imbalance. At least I have personally experienced the miracles that can come out of good operations research, or health systems research, whatever you want to call it. I think it is high time that we got ourselves a special programme for operations research on district health systems and I would propose to you to reflect, before you get together in the Executive Board or next year's Assembly, that we ought to have such a programme with strong extrabudgetary support to do much more research and development in this field.

To finish, Mr President, one more vital quality of your Organization is its transparency. It is that transparency which has attracted so many who are interested in being supportive of world health. Very often these were previously considered outsiders. Now we have collaborating centres by the thousands, and scientists inside these collaborating centres by the tens of thousands, who are eagerly working together in order to add to our knowledge about how to cope with making a better health world. Nongovernmental organizations have for the first time seen you open up the doors to them; they are still a little bit timid because they are not so sure you really want them to get inside the temple of WHO. We have asked and challenged the universities to try timidly to come in through the doors of WHO and see that they can benefit from their WHO too. I repeat my invitation to the universities to come closer to their WHO. And, after years of hesitation, we are finally getting at our colleagues and various health associations — the doctors, the nurses and many other health professionals. They are beginning to feel that they can afford to swing together with their WHO; and that, I think, is a tremendously hopeful opening for the future. They are all vital partners in our great health adventure. When I reflect on how governments, nongovernmental organizations, community cooperatives, these associations of health professionals, consumer representatives, industry, and you mention it, all of them, are increasingly inside our WHO temple and trying to be helpful, sometimes creating problems for us, but basically all wanting the same, namely to try to give support so that we can push our value system and health for all forward. I am very, very grateful to that evolution and I only hope that it can be speeded up over the coming years.

Mr President, I hope then I have said enough to show that WHO remains, in our contemporary world, highly relevant. In my humble opinion, when you look at the rather sordid international scenario, WHO is one of its redeeming features and it is your responsibility to keep WHO that way. It is your responsibility to make sure that the health momentum your Organization has generated continues to increase, and that the enthusiasm it has generated throughout the world does not burn itself out. Only the mythical bird, the phoenix, burnt itself out and then arose with new vitality from the ashes. WHO is not a mythical bird; it is a solid reality. If you therefore act as guardians of its moral values and the policies that emanate from these values, if you do that you know very well in your hearts and minds that you will ensure that your Organization remains a solid, highly relevant reality, leading people everywhere in the world to better health in the year 2000 and way beyond.

Remarks by Dr H. Nakajima, Director-General Elect, to the World Health Assembly, 4 May 1988

Mr President, distinguished delegates, it is not easy for me to find words to adequately express my feelings on being elected Director-General of the World Health Organization by the Forty-first World Health Assembly. I am deeply moved by the confidence you show in me by this act and the honour which you bestow on me personally and on my country as well.

But it is also no less an honour to the Member States of the Western Pacific and South-East Asia Regions and to my colleagues there with whom I have had the privilege to work over the past nine years. Equally important, it is a vindication of the democratic process that the World Health Organization has the good fortune to enjoy.

The World Health Organization has emerged from the scrutiny which is being cast on all the United Nations system and has been judged as one which is doing a good job and moving in the right direction. This surely reflects the correctness of our common goals, the wisdom of our policy-makers, the dedication and loyalty of our staff, the inspired leadership of our past Directors-General, particularly Dr Halfdan Mahler, the commitment of the Regional Directors, and the steadfast support and cooperation of all our Member States.

In accepting the position of Director-General I am inspired by the achievements of WHO in the 40 years of its existence. I am also influenced by my own experience as a young man in Japan, growing up amidst the misery and tragedy of war in contrast to the prosperity and development that have been achieved in the years of peace which have followed. It has strengthened my conviction that the pathway to social development is directly related to our success in maintaining peace in the world. I have lived half my life outside the country of my birth and this experience will certainly help me to discharge my responsibilities over the next five years in a manner worthy of the trust you have shown in me.

I am mindful of the challenges which lie ahead.

We live in fragile times. The gap between the "haves" and "have nots" has not narrowed. If we, Member States and WHO, are to achieve our goal of health for all in the spirit of social equity we must establish new partnerships and engage in different dialogues involving the world community — not only with North—South but also East—West participants. But our dialogues must be followed by concerted and timely action. Talk alone is no longer enough.

Even before we win our battle against the communicable diseases which has engaged us since our earliest days, many countries must now, in addition, face the burden of aging and the chronic and degenerative diseases. At the same time still too many people in the world live without the benefit of safe drinking-water and sanitation. And with each passing day threats to the environment from man-made pollution make more tenuous our very survival. On top of these sad recitations we are more recently assailed by a new and terrible disease — AIDS — for which there is as yet no cure.

The solution to any of these problems would tax the resources of even the rich countries but, sad to say, in the midst of these realities, world economic recovery is slow and remains uncertain.

But there are encouraging signs about us that our common desire for peace may soon be achieved. I am optimistic that this will result in more resources being channelled towards health and social development and will lead us closer to our goal of health for all.

In all humility I pledge to you that I shall spare no effort to maintain the proud image of your Organization. With the continuing support of all of you, our Member States, working as equals in the spirit of friendly cooperation,

we, the WHO Secretariat, with the strongest support of the regional directors, dedicate ourselves to achieving our common health goals. In so doing,
we shall surely be leading the World Health Organization towards even
greater excellence and making our own contribution to world peace.

Technical Discussions on Leadership Development for Health for All, 5-7 May 1988

The background of the Technical Discussions

Leadership is a concept covering the human dimension of activities that initiate and foster the process of change. Leadership development for health for all is a new initiative which has no precedent. The subject is challenging and complex. Essential to the issues is the development of leadership and the nature and cultivation of the vision, values and leadership skills of individuals who are in a position to mobilize others.

The Technical Discussions on the topic "Leadership development for health for all" were held on 5-7 May 1988 under the Chairmanship of Dame Nita Barrow, Permanent Representative of Barbados to the United Nations, New York.

The goal of health for all by the year 2000 is a vision founded on social equity, on the urgent need to reduce the gross inequalities in the health status of people in the world. It is a vision whose range of view encompasses fundamental change in the way health is perceived, promoted, protected, and provided. These changes represent a fundamental shift in values of all those involved. They include:

- change in how people, individually, take greater responsibility for the protection and promotion of their health;
- change in the way people participate collectively in health;
- change in the perception and value systems of the health providers, in which involving and empowering of people assume greater importance;
- change in the organization and administration of the health system, emphasizing bottom-up planning, delegating power, creating alliances of support and developing new partnerships; and
- change in the attitude and perception of the policy/decision-makers, characterized by greater concern for social equity.

These perceived changes are embodied in the Global Strategy for Health for All by the Year 2000 through primary health care, which was unanimously adopted by the Member States of the World Health Organization in 1981.

A clear understanding of the critical issues affecting the implementation of national strategies and courageous and imaginative initiatives to resolve these issues adequately by those in leadership positions in health and health-related fields were also considered imperative. Recognizing this need, the Director-General of WHO launched a new initiative in January 1985, called "Health-for-All Leadership Development". The initiative is based on the premise that the implementation gap could be substantially narrowed if individuals in leadership positions understood more fully the process involved in developing and implementing the strategy for health for all, pursued its values, and developed within themselves the appropriate qualities and abilities to lead the process.

The principal aim of the initiative is to create (or mobilize) a critical mass of people in each country who are in a position to motivate others and direct their national health development processes towards the goal of health for all.

In order to address the key question "how can leadership that can generate a collective force in society to achieve the common goal of health for all through primary health care be developed", the Executive Board of WHO, at its seventy-eighth session in May 1986, decided that the subject of the Technical Discussions in 1988 would be "Leadership development for health for all".

The Discussions focused on clarifying the leadership functions required to initiate change within national situations in response to the challenge posed by health for all through primary health care and in dealing with crucial implementation issues. The process of leadership development within the national and international contexts was also explored. Specifically the Discussions evolved around three major questions:

- Why is leadership needed for health for all?
- What can leadership do in support of health for all?
- How can leadership be developed/enhanced?

The Technical Discussions were opened by the General Chairman, Dame Nita Barrow, on Thursday, 5 May 1988. There were some 400 participants including eminent leaders from many walks of life in different countries and from various sectors, international organizations, agencies, institutions and nongovernmental organizations, representing all levels of society — from the policy decision-making to the community.

The opening plenary session was followed by a Panel of speakers consisting of, in addition to the General Chairman and Dr H. Mahler, the Director-General of WHO, Dr C. Aurenche, Project Leader, Tokombéré, Cameroon; Professor J. Bryant, Aga Khan University, Pakistan; Dr A. Fakhro, Minister of Education, Bahrain; Dr M. Kökeny, Deputy Minister for Social Welfare and Health, Hungary; Dr E. Mohs, Minister of Health, Costa Rica; Professor O. Ransome-Kuti, Minister of Health, Nigeria; and Dr P. Senanayake, Assistant Secretary-General, IPPF. The panel was moderated by Professor J. Michael, Dean, School of Public Health, University of Hawaii, USA.

The speakers represented different levels and dimensions of leadership and, drawing on their personal experiences, highlighted a number of key issues and challenges for accelerating health development, as an "appetizer" for subsequent group discussions. Highlights of the panel discussion included: the leadership vacuum and crisis; health for all as a vehicle to challenge the present social climate of amorality; the need to generate leadership that included empowering communities to become full partners in health development; some of the essential leadership attributes for health for all; the impact strong policy leadership could make to improving the health status through primary health care; and the special contribution educational institutions could make to leadership development.

Report of Dame Nita Barrow, General Chairman of the Technical Discussions, to the World Health Assembly, 9 May 1988 (Extracts)

I am honoured and privileged to present to this distinguished gathering — this galaxy of health leaders — the report of the Technical Discussions on the exciting and challenging subject: "Leadership Development for Health for All".

The positive force of the sense of involvement, together with the feeling of personal challenge and commitment, prevailed during this period throughout the many halls and rooms of these buildings in which we met.

I would compare what was happening in the groups to fibres of cloth absorbing a dye, as the participants became more and more imbued with the vital necessity of developing leadership.

We have just about reached the midpoint between the time we made the historical decision to achieve health for all through primary health care and the turn of the century, the year 2000.

That political commitment made by us in 1978 was based on a vision that foresaw the reduction of inequalities in both health and health care among the people we are privileged to serve. A vision — not a mere dream — and not wishful thinking: but a vision based on proven facts furnished by the pioneering leadership of many countries and of groups within countries.

Now, 10 years later, we must summon the courage to challenge ourselves as to whether we measure up to the covenant of that agreement. And that is an essential quality of leadership itself — to be able to recognize our successes as well as to face up to our failures — to learn from them, capitalize on them, and move forward with an even greater determination and enthusiasm towards the vision in which we truly believe.

There was a general consensus that, in the world today, we are facing a vacuum, some went as far as to use the term "crisis" of leadership — leadership which generates a social conscience, which is concerned with the prevailing social injustices that, I might add, have even increased in all of our societies. This is what Dr Mahler refers to when he emphasizes the need for "moral leadership".

Some of us who had been involved in the health for all movement since the beginning thought that the principles of primary health care provided the force or the vehicle for generating this moral leadership, starting within the smallest communities and reaching through the highest national and international levels. We took it for granted that this message was clearly projected in the Declaration of Alma-Ata on primary health care. History proved that we were wrong.

Now, ten years after Alma-Ata, it seems that perhaps we took too much for granted — that even though we have made some progress pursuing the course, the fundamental principles of the Declaration have not been either fully understood or "internalized" — that there is a sizeable gap between our commitment at Alma-Ata and what was done back home. It has also become evident that managerial or technocratic approaches alone will not get us to our goals. Primary health care, above all, must become a social movement — a movement in which people in all walks of life are involved as active partners and not just as passive recipients of the so-called benefits. It is a movement which is not restricted to the extension of services, but aims first and foremost at expanding responsibilities for health from the individual level right up to the top policy level. A difficult concept for us to grasp, especially for those of us who are used to top-down thinking.

Such social movements demand leadership at all levels, thereby sharing the vision of health for all and reflecting certain essential qualities.

And what are these "essential qualities"? First and foremost, having a social conscience which generates a genuine concern for social injustices. Further, a social movement such as primary health care cannot be dependent upon a single charismatic leader. (No offence meant, Dr Mahler.) It requires a collective leadership, encompassing all levels of society, creating a collective "force" towards the goal. Nor can it be limited within ministries of health or the health sector, but must comprise other sectors: academic circles, health professionals and above all members of the community. The role of the nongovernmental organizations is particularly important.

It must be an enabling and empowering type of leadership which believes in the inherent strength and ability of the people, thereby building self-reliance. It must be a sharing leadership in which there is no monopolizing of power (very difficult for us to accept). In other words, such leadership must re-endorse the values and principles of primary health care.

Of course, credibility is important. People must believe in such leadership. And the credibility must be earned by working with people, listening to them, taking on responsibilities which are larger and outside oneself, dealing with problems and situations with which the people are concerned, and overcoming obstacles and resistance.

This requires a balance between moral and social values, attitudes, and the ability to identify needs and solve problems, and to manage change, the latter most important of all.

Among the more critical functions of such leadership are: raising awareness and concern for the issues of equity and social justice in society as a whole, building and expanding partnerships and new alliances for support of health universally, and communicating on health issues. There seems to be concern that people working in health are generally poor communicators, which calls for drastic changes in the situation. And there is also the issue of the moral and social responsibility of the media.

Consensus was reached in the discussions that while leadership was needed "across the board", leadership at the community level represented the most powerful potential to accelerate momentum towards the goal of health for all. And in this context, it was noted that women and youth groups could play a highly significant role. There were youth present in the Discussions who shared their thoughts and ideas and showed what role they could play.

In response to the question: "Can we develop or foster such leadership?" the overwhelming response was: "yes!". And this was true not only for those of us who are in leadership positions at many different levels in the health system, but also for the new generation of leaders. But there are prerequisites which must be recognized and met.

Our working and educational environments must be conducive to creating and promoting moral leadership. Opportunities must exist to exercise leadership — to innovate, to challenge the often outmoded systems which hinder rather than facilitate progress. And it was recognized that there were many barriers in our work environments and in our educational institutions. Although capable managers and academicians are present, they do not always possess the leadership qualities I have touched upon earlier. They will be the first to recognize this.

It is evident that both social conscience and moral values must appear early in life if they are to be built-in personal ingredients. Therefore, leadership development must begin in primary schools. Furthermore, higher learning institutions, particularly for health professionals, require major modification which would allow students to learn in the communities and from the communities, by working with them.

Several practical recommendations have evolved from these Technical Discussions. These apply to individuals, governments, nongovernmental organizations, educational institutions, and WHO.

The principal message is that, at all levels, the values inherent in the primary health care approach need to be "internalized". The real message ingrained in these values must be clearly understood by all. These values are about involving, enabling and empowering people, first and foremost. They are about creating and fostering the environment and conditions which facilitate the involvement of people creatively in assuming greater responsibility for their own health and for the health of their communities. They are about developing partnerships — new partnerships, which, in turn, require new mechanisms. Therefore, it is very important that these recommendations be carefully studied and *then* put into practice — NOT left on a piece of paper.

Recommendations to WHO call for continuing and sustained support at all levels for this promising initiative, in order for it to become a self-perpetuating, a self-generating movement. This is required at every level, from the village to the global level. Each level must create its own mechanism to develop and support leadership and to assess its effectiveness in achieving the primary health care goals.

We also felt that leadership for health for all through primary health care is a personal challenge and implies a personal commitment. We therefore made a Declaration of such commitment, adopting a five-point personal agenda for action.

These Technical Discussions signify an historic landmark, in assessing and evaluating whether we leaders can be and have been converted to primary health care.

Ten years ago, in Alma-Ata, we made a *political commitment* to achieve health for all through primary health care. Today, we are making *a personal commitment* towards this challenge. We are convinced that leadership development for health for all is an imaginative and courageous initiative, which provides new opportunities to inform and communicate, to expand partnership among people, to empower people to take on new responsibilities for their health, the health of their families, and of their communities.

It is my personal responsibility to call upon this august assembly to unanimously adopt this Declaration of Personal Commitment,[1] so that it truly becomes a personal challenge to all, and not just another piece of paper. I urge its widest dissemination — every health and community worker should have it. Every health facility should display it. It must become a collective force which will generate the momentum we need to realize our vision — the vision of the goal of health for all through primary health care. Dr Mahler, our personal commitment is also a commitment to carry on the vision of health for all which you have initiated and advanced and to see that it is taken to its ultimate conclusion. I am sure that your successor, Dr H. Nakajima, will carry the vision forward.

---

[1] The Health Assembly adopted a resolution on leadership development for health for all (see Annex 2). The Declaration of Personal Commitment was annexed to that resolution.

Round Table Debate on the tenth anniversary of Alma-Ata, 9 May 1988 (Extracts)

Introduction

The key event of the 1988 World Health Assembly in relation to Alma-Ata was the Round Table Debate, chaired by Sir John Reid, extracts of which are given here. The purpose of the Round Table was to capture the spirit of the Alma-Ata conference through reflections by those who were there in 1978, and also to share the perceptions of others about important developments that have taken place since Alma-Ata, including the many problems and issues that remain to be addressed.

The participants in the Round Table reflected the regional organization of WHO and the international and nongovernmental organizations that participate with WHO in the health for all effort:

Dr M. Adhyatma (Indonesia) for the South-East Asia Region
Dr A.R. Al-Awadi (Kuwait) for the Eastern Mediterranean Region
Dame Nita Barrow, on behalf of nongovernmental organizations
Dr John H. Bryant, Rapporteur, Riga Meeting
Dr Marcella Davies, WHO Representative, Kenya
Dr N. Gay (Bahamas) for the Region of the Americas
Mr J. Grant, Executive Director, UNICEF
Dr W. Koinange (Kenya) for the African Region
Dr H. Mahler, Director-General, WHO
Dr N. Sadik, Executive Director, UNFPA
Sir John Reid (*Moderator*)
Professor Oleg P. Ščepin, First Deputy Minister of Health, Chief Delegate of the USSR
Dr S. Tapa (Tonga) for the Western Pacific Region
Professor B. Westerholm (Sweden) for the European Region

SIR JOHN REID:

In 1974 the World Health Assembly reviewed the Director-General's Report for 1973 as well as the Fifth Report on the World Health Situation. The Assembly noted the marked disparities in health and in health services between countries, and it asked the Director-General to report on what could be done to secure more effective coordination between WHO's activities and national health programmes. The Director-General submitted the requested report to the Executive Board in January 1975. The Board in its turn emphasized that priority attention should be given to primary health care at the community level. And in transmitting the Director-General's report to the Assembly, the Board suggested that there should be a review of the experience of countries in providing primary health care.

The 1975 Assembly asked the Executive Board to arrange an international conference on the subject. Invitations were forthcoming from several countries and the 1976 Assembly agreed to accept the invitation from the USSR, at the same time gladly accepting the generous offer of UNICEF to cosponsor the event.

Next in chronology, the World Health Assembly of 1977 clearly reaffirmed WHO's constitutional objectives and came to the now well-known conclusion that the main social target of governments and WHO in the coming decades should be the attainment by all citizens of the world by the year 2000 of a level of health that would permit them to lead a socially and economically productive life.

That aspiration was interpreted by the Executive Board at its meeting in January 1978 as an acceptable level of health for all and therefore it passed into general parlance as health for all by the year 2000.

The scene was now set for the Alma-Ata Conference on Primary Health Care, which took place in September 1978 and was attended by delegations from 134 Member States and by representatives of 67 United Nations organizations, specialized agencies and nongovernmental organizations in official relations with WHO and UNICEF. The Conference had been preceded by a series of national, regional, and international meetings on primary health care, the outcomes of which were fed into the Alma-Ata proceedings. The main documentation for the Conference, however, was the joint report by the Director-General of WHO and the Executive Director of UNICEF, simply entitled "Primary Health Care" — a document which is well known to all of you and which, in only 133 paragraphs, sets out a comprehensive agenda for the definition and establishment of primary health care.

Ten years ago, the Alma-Ata Conference and the entire world first heard the Declaration of Alma-Ata from the lips of Dr Marcella Davies. So it is both fitting and delightful that she should now be invited to repeat it to this audience.

(At this point Dr Davies read out the Declaration)

At Alma-Ata, the President of the Conference was the then Minister of Health of the USSR, Professor Boris Petrovskii, the distinguished surgeon. In his opening speech Professor Petrovskii referred to the treasure-house of world experience in health matters relevant to the work of the Conference, and to the many useful principles, methods and techniques which, if drawn upon, could help to achieve the desired ends of primary health care more rapidly.

It is now appropriate that we should hear the thoughts of Professor Oleg Ščepin, First Deputy Minister of Health of the USSR, whose Kazakh SSR hosted the Alma-Ata Conference and whose Latvian SSR hosted a subsequent meeting at Riga some weeks ago.

PROFESSOR ŠČEPIN:

Ten years have elapsed now since the time when the unprecedented Alma-Ata Conference on Primary Health Care, organized by the World Health Organization and UNICEF, unanimously adopted its final document, which has become the guideline for achieving health care at all levels — global and national — in order to achieve the final goal of health for all. The Declaration and recommendations of that document have echoed throughout the world. The content of the document was supported not only at the Thirty-second and subsequent World Health Assemblies but also by the Thirty-fourth General Assembly of the United Nations, which approved the Declaration of Alma-Ata and called on all the Member States to apply the measures put forward in it.

In March of this year a meeting was held in Riga, where it was unanimously recognized that the Declaration of Alma-Ata retains its relevance at the present time and up to the year 2000, and that primary health care remains the key element in the strategy for achieving health for all. We can say quite categorically that the link between health and socioeconomic development and the need for a comprehensive approach to solving most problems in the field of health are more and more widely acknowledged in all the countries of the world.

However, it is also becoming clearer that high political commitments are not a guarantee of good results, and without a progressive socioeconomic policy in the interest of the populations of various countries, we are unlikely to see any substantial progress in realizing the concept of health for all.

There is still a lack of financial, material and personnel resources, and these problems are often exacerbated by the fact that many donor countries, basing themselves on their own political and social interests, prefer to invest their resources in specific vertical programmes with an autonomous structure to achieve immediate results and not in development of integrated long-term programmes for developing general health infrastructure based on primary health care which, in the final analysis, would promote the ability of the country to become self-sufficient and independent.

The participants at the Riga meeting also noted that achieving health for all remains a permanent goal for all nations and will go beyond the year 2000, and called on all countries to intensify their activities in the social and economic spheres in order to secure financial resources and policies needed to achieve health for all, bringing in nongovernmental organizations, the public at large, and also the interested sectors of the population in a spirit of cooperation.

The last 10 years have demonstrated that our Organization and its Member States have achieved a great deal of progress. We can say categorically that, in spite of the many financial difficulties encountered by the Organization over the last few years, it has been able to overcome them and it has achieved some of its humanitarian goals with its Global Strategy for Health for All by the

Year 2000. This is due to the great authority exercised by the World Health Organization and to the trust that Member States have in it.

SIR JOHN REID:

I have invited three of those who were at Alma-Ata, from where they sit, just to reflect on how they recall the spirit of that meeting. And the first person I would invite to do so is Dame Nita Barrow.

DAME NITA BARROW:

Who could forget Alma-Ata? Perhaps, for those of us in the Christian Medical Commission, the joy was working with both the World Health Organization and UNICEF in the preparation for Alma-Ata. Never before had nongovernmental organizations been given their rightful place as the people who really knew what was happening — they were the organizations in the field who were the first to attack the innovative approaches to health care. Alma-Ata itself, you've already described its beauty, the surprising friendliness of its people, the atmosphere that was created both in the great hall and in the beautiful Pushkin Library where we met for informal discussions.

DR BRYANT:

I was struck by the boldness of the attempt to discuss a subject with such far-reaching implications so seriously by such experienced people. There was a gradual awareness among many of us that this was no ordinary international conference, that something special was happening. This was brought home forcefully by the Director-General's speech when he asked the now famous eight questions. He said, in 1978 at Alma-Ata, that it is very important to reach an understanding on the principles of primary care and on the actions that will have to be taken to be sure that it is properly understood and systematically introduced and strengthened throughout the world so that — and here's the point — so that it becomes a living reality whose implementation no reactionary health forces can ever stop.

I'll read just two of the eight questions: Are you ready to make preferential allocations of health resources to the social periphery as an absolute priority? Are you ready to fight the political and technical battles required to overcome any social and economic obstacles and professional resistance to the universal introduction of primary health care?

It was at this time that many of us recognized that there was a farsightedness at work, a distance vision involved. And we realized that we were involved in something truly historic. Now, in retrospect, we know that.

DR TAPA:

All the participants in the Alma-Ata conference were people belonging to one family — the human family — getting together to discuss and decide on the future course of one of the fundamental human rights — the health of every human being and collectively the health of mankind, without distinction of race, religion, political belief, or economic or social condition. The

result of the Conference is now history. The priceless Declaration of Alma-Ata is a legacy that we pass on to the future generations of mankind.

SIR JOHN REID:

The first subject that the panel might address themselves to is the simple question "Did Alma-Ata really make a difference?"

MR GRANT:

The answer to that question clearly has to be "yes". At a meeting in Talloires a few weeks ago we were discussing the remarkable progress of recent years on the child health front, using primary health care principles. Barber Conable, President of the World Bank, asked the question, "What about the application of these same principles to other fields — education, food production?" The reply I had to give was that in these other fields there is no comparable doctrine that focuses on reaching the great mass of people. It is within the doctrine of Alma-Ata that it has been possible to push forward with the kind of breakthroughs we've had. We don't have that in education. UNESCO has not brought about on its side a comparable over-arching framework. Neither has the FAO on food for people.

So I would argue very forcefully that several million children were alive last year who would not have been alive if it had not been for the momentum developed within the framework provided by Alma-Ata.

The other side of the question "Did Alma-Ata make a difference?" is to say, "yes, but not sufficiently so". Because if it were making a sufficient difference you would not have the equivalent of two Hiroshimas of children dying every week from largely preventable causes.

PROFESSOR WESTERHOLM:

Did Alma-Ata make a difference? Yes, but changes take time and many of us are impatient. One can look at this as involving four phases. The first started with Alma-Ata and has spread like rings on water. In the establishment of the targets for health for all in a majority of European countries you can find the ideas, legislation and political will. You can see it elaborated into national strategies and down to county/municipality level. Now we are in the second phase, that of implementation, which is much more difficult; we find obstacles which sometimes we feel are insurmountable, but have to be overcome. We have now to sort ourselves out and define these obstacles and how to overcome them in order to come into the third phase, when everything is more stabilized, and then into the fourth, where we have success. I believe we will have success but we have to work hard for it.

DR ADHYATMA:

What happened after Alma-Ata? Confusion. Confusion about what? The meaning of primary health care. What does it mean? For some people it is just an extension of the existing health care delivery system. For another group, primary health care is a second-quality health care delivery system. For still another group, primary health care is health care for the poor people. And for another group, primary health care is the first contact between the patient and the health worker. Gradually people started to understand the meaning of primary health care correctly and gradually the primary health care approach was accepted and high-level political commitment was obtained in many countries of the South-East Asia Region.

Both health for all and primary health care have taken root and are starting to have their effect. What is the effect in the South-East Asia Region? Let me talk about indicators — indicators of success. There has been a significant decline in infant mortality in the Region with four countries having succeeded in reducing their infant mortality rate below 50 per 1000 live births. Another proof of the success of primary health care is the coverage with services. Among these services, coverage of the Expanded Programme on Immunization has increased to 80% from being very low. This shows that the primary health care approach is taking root in this Region.

DR KOINANGE:

Did Alma-Ata make a difference? The answer is a big "yes". This was an opportunity for governments and nongovernmental organizations to help communities to change their approach to health. It was in fact an invitation to all these groups to demystify the approaches they have always taken towards their own health. When one looks at what has happened to these agencies in the last ten years, there has been very good change.

I particularly would like to mention that the former advisory/donor/recipient approach, which had always characterized the things that we had known in health, has changed. In one particular country I have seen an excellent relationship between the World Health Organization and UNICEF in that we have been able to go out together in the field and have been really close partners in establishing primary health care.

DR AL-AWADI:

The Alma-Ata Declaration represented a revolution in concepts and ideas. These concepts have sought to stress the fact that health is an individual and personal matter and is not only to be left in the hands of doctors. Health was deemed to be a comprehensive, total, community movement and a complete endeavour that started from the level of education, the improvement of sewerage, the provision of appropriate drinking-water supplies, appropriate housing, the provision of sound food and nutrition — that is to say, all those basic concepts that together represent health. This is an old concept for the developed world because most of the countries of the developed world live in a degree of prosperity where all such services are available. But when we started trying to achieve these goals in the developing countries we found that it was not an easy task. It represented an overwhelming comprehensive social movement that required the establishment of the health notion in its wider sense.

The Alma-Ata Declaration is the real revolution that enables us to restore genuine concepts in the activities of our Organization. This Organization in

the past had lost its way and steered away from the main path of its work; it had sought to tackle individual diseases or develop health services in isolation from one another. It had forgotten that health is a comprehensive movement or action which starts and ends with the individual. And without this concept I do not believe we can achieve a better world for the individual.

DR SADIK:

Alma-Ata was a historic and trail-blazing conference. It set a pattern for collaboration, with health not just the responsibility of the health ministry but of every nation-building department in a country. And, most importantly, the individual was responsible for his or her own health. Underlying all these concepts was the need to mobilize resources of all kinds — financial, human, technical and political.

In achievements, infant mortality has declined tremendously and fertility levels have gone down but, surprisingly, maternal mortality remains as high and as horrible as ever. Considering that part of this concept of primary health care has really emerged from the maternal and child health care sector, the fact that maternal mortality remains so high is something that must concern us very much.

DR GAY:

Has Alma-Ata made a difference? Yes, yes, it has. Ten years later we must say that this conceptual framework, this social development declaration must stand at the very top of accomplishments by any international organization.

It has been with reason and not without emotion that we have set about carrying out the objectives of Alma-Ata. Yes, a deliberate attempt to change the course of health development; a conscious, collective effort to influence in a favourable direction the health of our peoples. And has it made a difference? In spite of falling income per head, in spite of decreasing personal income, in spite of decreased government spending in many instances, the Region of the Americas set up quantifiable measures of health that make it possible today, after ten years, to look back and to say that we have seen some good things happen.

Eighteen of our countries have attained the goal of reducing infant mortality to 30 per 1000: 80% of all of our children are immunized against the scourges of childhood diseases; we have safe drinking-water for an appreciable number of both our rural and urban populations; we have adequate sanitation for a vastly increased number of people; equity in health; the coverage of our people; the availability of services. We have seen this reach some 270 million people.

DAME NITA BARROW:

I regret that I come after my colleague from the same Region, because I'm going to be dissident. The poorest of the poor in our Region are still not being reached, even in the developed countries. I am amazed that countries that would say they have the resources have not attacked their real problems. If there are 40 000 homeless people in a city, then we are not providing primary health care. If we still have a high mortality rate for mothers in some countries, that is not acceptable. I know that primary health care has reached many people — yes, it has made a difference — but we must not be euphoric. We must look at the fact that even the health professionals have lulled themselves to sleep by saying, "The first level of care is primary care".

We have said we can provide more hospital beds and we are giving a bigger percentage of our total budget to health. That is still not primary care. As long as we have not gone into the communities, then we have not gone far enough. All we can say is that we have started on a very long journey and the end is not yet in sight.

SIR JOHN REID:

Yes, it has made a difference, but one has to say that always in a qualified way. And it has made a difference to all types of countries, developed countries as well as developing countries. But there has been no self-satisfaction and there has been a clear desire to explore where we go.

I would like to touch upon one important issue, that is the question of people. Do people in health know what we're about?

DR AL-AWADI:

I want to deal with the role of doctors and health workers. To what extent do they understand these concepts? I believe that this is a basic problem. Those people, regretfully, are not trained in such concepts in colleges and universities, and naturally we cannot expect such people to expand these concepts among the public. The public always looks to these leaders in health care as a source of information — a source of correct concepts. I believe that people can understand these concepts, but until now we have not reached people in the right way. The true path is to focus more intensively on health in life rather than just disease, because healthy living is the basis of health.

DR ADHYATMA:

How much do health professions really know about primary health care? Most health workers in most of the developing countries were not trained or educated to implement the primary health care approach. They were trained to treat sick people. So there must be a change in their attitude, and to be able to change it we have to change also the curricula in the nursing schools and universities. Nurses and doctors have to be trained not only in curative skills but particularly in prevention and in promotion of health. They also have to be trained to communicate, to organize people, to organize the community. So if we would like to accelerate primary health care then one of the major things to do is to change the attitudes of the health workers.

DR KOINANGE:

There is no doubt that the weakest link we have is that our health professionals do not yet know about the concept of primary health care.

117

To go to another subject, in the future we are going to depend on young people and the information on primary health care should be beamed at the youth of the world, and also at women, who are very good participants in primary health care.

DR MAHLER:

I was with two African statesmen in the last few months and both of them said: "We want to have primary medical care for our rural people". And I can assure you when I tried to figure out what they meant by that, it was medicine, medicine, medicine in a good old conventional medical Western sense. Quite clearly what we tried to go for in Alma-Ata was to get out of the confusion that medicine is synonymous with health. That has to do with people called health professionals — they never were health professionals; they are medical professionals, all of them. The ministries of health have never had anything to do with health, they are ministries of medicine. So it is not surprising that somehow we don't have any kind of impact or penetration when it comes to the professionals being involved.

All of these groups, from the politicians to the professionals to the leaders down the hierarchical ladder, all of them have great expertise in cannibalism, that is, they are eating their people and they pretend they can represent them. But, as we well know, it is very tough to represent the people you have eaten!

The Chinese have a proverb which really expresses what people's participation is all about: "You go to the people, you live with them, you learn from them and you love them". If you can't do that you will never get people's participation.

DR SADIK:

Reflecting on Alma-Ata ten years ago, I believe that it would be unthinkable today to hold an Alma-Ata with just WHO, UNICEF and the nongovernmental organizations as participants. Surely there would have to be the involvement of UNDP, the World Bank, UNFPA, among others, as decisive partners or participants in the whole process. Furthering the goals of Alma-Ata can be hastened or helped if you broaden the base for the support of the Alma-Ata objectives. I say this for a couple of reasons: one is that **what was sought at Alma-Ata was to mobilize resources from all avenues and to make health an integral, key component of development.** Not that health should be a by-product of economic development; not that health should be given as something that a government grants to its people. Health is a right and a key element of development. Without it development will not take place. I don't think that the ministries of health can achieve this by themselves. We need to mobilize even more resources for this purpose by involving ministries of finance, planning, and so forth.

This is why WHO and UNICEF should consider enlarging the number of organizations that they invite to participate in the promotion of health for all by the year 2000. In this way you can get the participation and involvement of a lot more people because these organizations have direct links with many other population groups. The idea is not just for health groups or people who are ill to participate in community and health promotion, but for all people to participate.

DR BRYANT:

I would like to say a word in favour of the capacity of community people to take care of their own problems. In the squatter settlements of urban Karachi we have primary health care programmes. They have identified serious malnutrition among children as a very important cause of death. We also learned that we as doctors and nurses were almost helpless to improve the status of those malnourished children. It was not until the community women, whom we had recruited from houses and lanes, who were monitoring the children and following them day by day, it was not until they realized the problems and saw that we were failing, that they could take over and progress towards solving the problem. It was they who could convince mothers to feed their children differently.

Now some reflections about the discussions at Riga, where we reviewed successes and failures since Alma-Ata. We concluded that there is no doubt that health for all and primary health care have served the world well. At the same time, while there have been substantial gains in most countries, there has been a slowness and even stagnation of progress in many countries. If you look at projections for the year 2000, you will find a large number of African and South Asian countries where infant, young child and maternal mortality rates will still be at levels that the world must consider completely unacceptable. These are the Hiroshimas of which Jim Grant was speaking.

At Riga, we considered two types of problem as paradigms. These problems were thrown up to send certain signals to WHO and its Member States. One of those sets of problems was the continued high mortality rates in the least developed countries. The signal here is that even though we know the causes of those problems and what to do about them, the steps that have been taken in those countries have been inadequate to relieve the extreme suffering that those rates represent. We know the problems, we know what to do about them, but we have been unable to make progress that is substantial.

The second paradigm was that of population growth and ecological deterioration — that is, with continued population growth there is over-grazing, over-cutting, depletion of water tables, a slowly decreasing carrying capacity of ecological systems, decreasing agricultural productivity, decreasing income, then a stagnation of development and even an increase in mortality. This is an example of development-gone-wrong, a distortion of the expected development process. The signal here is that this is an entirely different kind of problem, one less familiar to the health sector, with no clear solutions; it calls for new analyses, new partners, new resources.

This was a turning point at Riga: the recognition that what is being done is not enough. As WHO turns the corner of the first decade after Alma-Ata it needs to ready itself for a new set of problems. Tomorrow will not be yesterday, and yesterday's answers, though they brought glory, will not serve tomorrow. So there was a call for new forms of analyses, new partnerships, new mechanisms of action and new resources.

The debate at Riga turned these issues over and over. The result was "Alma-Ata reaffirmed at Riga — A statement of renewed and strengthened commitment to health for all by the year 2000 and beyond.". But this was not simply a self-congratulatory exercise. There was an acknowledgement of the important shortfalls, that serious problems remained almost untouched by the health for all effort. New problems are emerging that are already defying solutions. To address this range of persisting and emerging problems, the meeting at Riga suggested a number of actions to be taken. Ten are listed, but I'll just mention a few by title: empowering people; strengthening district health systems based on primary care; overcoming problems that continue to resist solution; finally, a special priority initiative in support of the least developed countries.

The last point, about the least developed countries, is based on the fact that, while most countries have benefited from the health for all movement, a tragic residuum remains. These nations are not the causes of the problems of severe underdevelopment, they are the victims of it. They have been marginalized by it and, to a large extent, abandoned to it. The resources and processes involved in international development have failed these people, and health for all to date has failed them as well. And so a special initiative is proposed which should be strongly intersectoral in nature as well as long term. Finally, we believe that WHO should monitor the rate of progress, which should serve as an indicator of the resolve of WHO and the Member States to deal with this most fundamental of challenges, namely the needs of countries which, without effective help, will likely slip further down the spiral of development failure.

SIR JOHN REID:

Thank you very much for that. It confirms that Riga was certainly no exercise in self-satisfaction. Now, nearing the end of our time, I would like to ask members of the panel to indicate the areas where they feel special effort is required.

DR SADIK:

I want to make three points. First, to reiterate, I think WHO and UNICEF must broaden the base of support for the goal of health for all by the year 2000. Second, much more attention must be given to the health of women and to the role and status of women. Women are at the heart of the development process. They not only manage their households but they manage household resources. An educated woman is more likely to produce educated and well-nourished children than an uneducated woman. You know the old adage: educate a woman and you educate a nation. This means that women are accepted not just as income-earners and mothers, but for themselves, for their contribution to the whole of the development process. It is only when women can assert their rights and have the opportunity to participate in decision-making for themselves and for their children that there can be progress in all the fields of development, including health care.

Third, when Alma-Ata took place, the population of the world was 4 billion. Today it is over 5 billion. By the end of the century it will be over 6 billion people. More than three-quarters of them will be in the developing world. Most of the 900 million people who will be added between now and the year 2000 will be in the developing world. Attention has to be given to these numbers being added in the developing regions, particularly in the regions that are least able to cope, including the ecological consequences and the burden on development resources. Population policies need to be developed that strike a balance between the growing numbers, their use of resources, and the possibility for socioeconomic development — the international community should support individual governments in the attainment of these goals.

DR AL-AWADI:

I think Riga has summarized our feeling and our fears for the future of Alma-Ata. It has addressed itself properly to what has been going on and what should be done in the future. It is very important to have some practical global pointers as to how to go from there. Maybe in 10 years we will meet here again and like to know what has been done. I think the momentum has started right now for the Alma-Ata Declaration. It is important that we actually grasp this momentum and monitor it more closely than has been done in the past: not just a routine follow-up and routine discussion of what happened.

I suggest that what has been put forward as the permanence of health for all should have a board of trustees to look after it. The Declaration and its concepts are so great that they should not be treated lightly or dissipated by simple activities here and there. They are concepts that are going to percolate down to the grass roots. A board of trustees might be composed of international experts, nongovernmental organizations, international organizations, university experts. It is not for me to say exactly how it should be composed or how it should function, but **we need some kind of board that can meet maybe once every two years, not simply to report to the Health Assembly but a meeting that is set up specifically to ensure that we are achieving the great goal that we set for ourselves when we made the Declaration of Alma-Ata.**

Second, one thing that was said at Alma-Ata was: "**A general policy of independence, peace, détente, disarmament could and should release additional resources that could well be devoted to peaceful aims and in particular the acceleration of social and economic development of which primary care is an essential part.**" It is just a coincidence that about a month from now the two leaders of the world will meet again in the Soviet Union to address themselves to détente and peace. I feel that a declaration from this meeting should be sent to those people, that some of the money saved could serve this world through actions related to health and development.

SIR JOHN REID:

Thank you Dr Al-Awadi, and may I say this in relation to your remark about a board of trustees and the other suggestions that have come from you and others: this is a celebration, but it is also a part of the World Health Assembly, and I hope members of the Assembly, the Executive Board and the Secretariat will bear in mind the many suggestions which have come up here which will stand much more scrutiny and development.

DR GAY:

The Region of the Americas agrees with the conclusions arrived at in Riga, and in particular the statement: "It is as clear as crystal that current approaches will not break through the intractability of the most difficult problems". Our Region has initiated three basic programme priorities for transformation. First, the development of our health service infrastructure. This must happen, we must find the human resources, we must train them for efficient utilization. Secondly, we must respond to priority health problems where they affect our most vulnerable groups. Third, there is also the collection and coordination of knowledge and management of information so that decisions can be properly made.

We have started additional initiatives. In the Region of the Americas we have already decided that we should eradicate poliomyelitis by the year 1990, and, in conjunction with UNICEF and Rotary International, we are moving in that direction. In our Region we have come up with subregional groupings with initiatives where common health priorities between countries are formed into projects that can attract additional extrabudgetary funding. And today we have four such subregional programmes in place.

PROFESSOR WESTERHOLM:

In order to move forward, we have to mobilize the critical mass of people at all levels. A critical mass of leaders has to have certain qualifications. We talked about vitamin C deficiency yesterday; I also have a number of Cs which should characterize this critical mass of leaders. They have to be competent, know what they are talking about. They have to have courage to change. It's difficult. They have to be creative in order to find new solutions to overcome the obstacles. They have to be able to communicate what their aims are, and there has to be continuity and consistency. This is a long road to go, and you need continuity and consistency.

DR KOINANGE:

At Alma-Ata, we said that urgent action was required. Urgent action is still required and we must intensify our efforts far more with respect to all health training institutions. We should focus more on the mothers, on youth, and we should request WHO to review regularly, in conjunction with other agencies, the progress we are making.

SIR JOHN REID:

Another practical suggestion which I hope has been heard by all. I would now ask the Executive Director of UNICEF, Mr James Grant, our distinguished guest today, to give us his thoughts having heard this welter of goodwill and self-criticism.

MR GRANT:

This has clearly been a fascinating discussion. I would like to make several points. First, the key lesson of the past decade stands out. That is, that the insights of the Declaration of Alma-Ata can be trusted for practical guidance. The countries that have applied those principles have achieved spectacular results. The second lesson of the past decade is that, despite the validity of the Declaration, countries have been slow to move from rhetorical acceptance of primary health care to effective application. Third, we all agree that health for all and, if I may add a parochial twist, particularly for all children, by the year 2000 through primary health care is the right goal. But to achieve it will require far far greater political will to make primary health care an urgent national goal than exists today. Child mortality rates will need to be reduced over the next 12 years at twice the mortality reduction rates of recent decades and of the 1980s to date if the desired goal of halving child death rates between 1980 and the year 2000 is to be achieved, or an infant-mortality rate of 50 is to be attained in all countries. The gap between that goal and what is set forth in the charter here is the equivalent of 20 Hiroshimas a year. The question that I and my colleagues in UNICEF would ask of our colleagues in this room is straightforward: "Shouldn't we, who have contributed so much to create the capacity now within the world's hand, contribute more — whether collectively or in clusters or individually — to ensure that that capacity is not wasted?" That morality does keep pace with our ability to change the face of the twenty-first century. We know how. It doesn't cost a lot. What it takes is political will.

Shouldn't we insist far more vigorously than has any civilization to date that morality must march with capacity? Shouldn't we assert unequivocally that it is now unacceptable for so many millions of children, and mothers, to die needlessly from causes so readily preventable through primary health care? Shouldn't morality be brought into step with our new capacity to move forward with primary health care? Shouldn't we insist that the still massive death rates of children be placed along with slavery, colonialism, racism and apartheid, on the shelf reserved for those things which are simply no longer acceptable to humankind?

In this spirit, I do think the point made by Dr Al-Awadi is well taken, and I would hope there would be a resounding noise from this World Health Assembly to the Summit taking place at the end of this month, that the Summit, which is concerned with preventing future destruction, does say something about preventing the destruction that is taking place on such a massive and terrible scale every day. And that in speaking out on this subject they speak out specifically in endorsing the concept of the 1990 goals that we have before us of universal child immunization, oral rehydration therapy and the eradication of poliomyelitis.

One very important ingredient of the first Alma-Ata was that the NGOs participated. I was not there, but the ones I've talked to said that the NGOs provided that special stimulus — a special push to the Conference that added very significantly. It is clear to me that if we're going to get a new morality, something that makes it unconscionable for us not to apply the principles of

123

primary health care, it is going to be the nongovernmental organizations that will play the key role. It is they who are playing the key role on women, on environment, on peace, and on so many other subjects. But it is true also that almost all of us here belong to NGOs ourselves, and there is a key role that each of us with our disciplinary prestige and professionalism can add to NGOs to help them help us create the climate.

SIR JOHN REID:

For the last 15 years I have learned, sometimes to my cost, that the Director-General always has the last word. I call upon Dr Halfdan Mahler.

DR MAHLER:

I will make my last word, Sir John, what one delegate to the Health Assembly said in 1977 when health for all was discussed: that this whole concept touches the raw nerves of a sick health system. It sets the spiritual dimension and the moral basis for setting up healthy health systems. That, I think, is a very good conceptual clarification of what we were talking about in Alma-Ata and more recently in Riga. But how do we prevent the dogmas of today from becoming the doubts of tomorrow? **Our real problem, and one of the great dogmas or doctrines of Alma-Ata and Riga, and also here today, is that health is part of development. That social productivity is related to economic productivity. That this is a totally new paradigm for health and development.** Clearly we have totally failed by being as sectarian as we have been, a local club — UNICEF/WHO — with a little smattering of the NGOs screaming in the wings. We have started getting the nursing constituency on the track, or they are getting on track of their own volition. But certainly the medical profession is not by any means getting on the track, and in that respect we have utterly failed. In Europe, attempts are being made to get the medical associations to swing together with the concepts of Alma-Ata and we must do much more to get them to do so. In addition, we must get the universities to swing and thereby other sectors in their professional education, to understand what development is all about. By development I mean both industrialized and developing countries because certainly the industrialized countries could do with a spot of development too.

That leads me to a ringing endorsement that we need a broader constituency. There's no doubt about that. We have not succeeded in making the NGOs feel fully part of that broad constituency of the value system of primary health care and health for all. Not at all. They would like to become much more meaningful. Now whether the NGOs in their present form do really represent people or we have to look also for other kinds of groupings much closer to people, cooperatives of all kinds, is a matter that we should look at. But we do need a board of trustees or a policy platform, where the potential trends of this movement of health for all/primary health care are subjected to an audit function or trusteeship function. I have no doubt about it. And I think perhaps the Assembly might be willing to launch that kind of a challenge to the world at large. Had we had such a platform, we really could go to town in Moscow with the superpowers and their bosses, and really call their hypocrisy when they say that when they disarm then some of the money could go to development. We've never seen one single dollar of that. And it's about time that their bluff should be called. They are using that argument again and again in all of their speeches; that we would love to disarm so that we could have beautiful development on spaceship earth — we've never seen any result of that talk. So let us really challenge them when we can. But we need a broader constituency in order to win.

The last point, which is very very close to my heart, especially as I leave WHO, is that we must have an obsession, a moral obsession, about the least developed of the developing countries. They are missing out totally, as Jack Bryant said, in the development process. It is development-gone-wrong. They are marginalized in the cynical economic climate of the contemporary world. With the kind of platform we are talking about, with UNICEF and WHO together with UNFPA and other multilateral agencies, we can look at how we can address the problems of their predicament at this time in history. They must be brought on board in a real and true sense before the year 2000. It is indispensable not so that they survive in misery, but that they survive so their children can realize their physical, social and spiritual potential. This is where I feel very, very strongly that we have to move on, and that we have not been able to, we have not been willing to do so. All of us are paying lip service to the needs of these countries but nothing really has been done.

If we could make a real entry point into the development dilemma of these countries through health for all/primary health care, I think we could also challenge the other partners in development, and somehow shame them into saying that this cannot possibly go on if we have the minimum of morality on spaceship earth.

SIR JOHN REID:

Thank you very much indeed, Dr Mahler. The time has come for me to draw these proceedings to a close, and my first very agreeable task is to thank all members of the panel for making my task as moderator so very easy. I would also like to thank all those who have worked here and in countries worldwide to make the aspirations of Alma-Ata a reality. Our ceremony is over, the work goes on, the agenda changes, the job will never finish. So let us regard this afternoon's event not only as a celebration but also as a re-dedication to the high practical aims articulated and enunciated at Alma-Ata and reaffirmed at Riga. Thank you.

Farewell remarks by Dr H. Mahler, Director-General, to the World Health Assembly, 9 May 1988

Since this is the last occasion I shall have as your Director-General to address you, permit me a very few and very brief personal reflections, because it is at moments like this that memories of a lifetime flash through one's mind like dreams, startling in their vividness and seemingly unreal. But they were very, very real indeed. Combating tuberculosis on horseback in the remote rural areas of Ecuador and then on to many years in India, working with the people of that country, to take the fight against tuberculosis a gigantic step forward. And that was done through painstaking research on the spot, looking at the social and economic factors no less than the technical ones. And then, Eureka! The control of tuberculosis became possible through ambulatory care under the palm trees, making it more humane, and making it possible to incur enormous financial savings. Then on to Geneva to try to convince the world's best specialists and policy-makers, and at the same time to demonstrate that it pays off to maintain a probing mind. It pays off to dare to innovate in the face of conventional knowledge. And incidentally, as I mentioned a few days ago, the industrialized countries, out of this new knowledge in tuberculosis, made more money than they ever contributed to WHO. That struggle of yesterday has become the accepted practice of today, thanks exclusively to the international credibility given to it by your Organization, the World Health Organization.

And why do I reminisce? Certainly not to satisfy the ego of a departing Director-General. I do it simply to illustrate by one small personal example the enormous strength of WHO, and to relive the satisfaction of having been part of your wonderful organization for so long.

Your organization has reached new pinnacles — from being a rather small health forum of primarily the more privileged countries, to becoming a universal health cooperative, embracing virtually the whole of humanity. It has moved from supranational assistance to its Member States to genuine cooperation with them. It has displayed a remarkable degree of democratic management, combining worldwide consensus on policy with decentralized management down to its Member States themselves. It has set entirely new health goals in keeping with its own definition of health as a state of physical, social, mental and spiritual well-being and not merely the absence of disease or infirmity. And I suppose it cannot be stated often enough that outstanding among these goals has been the attainment of health for all by the year 2000. Two of the essential pillars of the strategy for attaining that goal were political commitment and people's involvement. You have established, you have fortified these pillars within the Organization itself. You have done that by vowing to reach that goal of health for all by means of a strategy on which you agreed by resounding consensus, and you and the people you represent have shared the joys and the sorrows of the struggle to attain a decent level of health for all people everywhere, in the spirit of social justice.

When I look back, in particular on these past 15 years as your Director-General, my happiest memories by far are the close ties I have felt I had with you. Not only here, but first and foremost in your countries, with the people in the villages and in the towns, with your health professionals, with your health and political leaders. That I have been able in some very, very small way to contribute to your efforts to improve the health of your people will always remain my supreme satisfaction.

I turn now to my successor, my good friend and colleague, Dr Nakajima. I extend to you my warmest congratulations, and my very best wishes. The burden is not so light. The responsibilities are quite heavy. The pressures and counter-pressures are quite often enormous. It all requires a lot of energy, a lot of courage, a lot of imagination, a lot of aggressive humility. But when you consider the benefits your endeavours can help to bring about for the people of this world, and not least for the underprivileged, you will agree with me it is worthwhile. It is very worthwhile.

The era in the history of your Organization with which I had the privilege to be closely associated was, in my opinion, a glorious one. One in which you gave the world a new hope, a new vision of health and well-being and a new understanding of how to reach it, and through it how to reach genuine human development and dignity. I thank you most sincerely, each and every one of you, for that unique privilege, and I thank you in particular for your patience with my impatient exhortations that your WHO should keep on doing more and doing better. I thank all the WHO staff everywhere most warmly and I wish you all, Member States and staff, I wish all of you the courage and the determination to make sure that this solid and yet so fragile Organization never looks back but moves inexorably forward into even more glorious eras. I thank you all.

To the year 2000 and beyond

The tasks before us

The meeting at Riga provided a careful review of the problems and prospects associated with Alma-Ata and health for all, and a series of proposals were then considered at the World Health Assembly. At the Assembly, further observations were made, during discussions of the working committees, at the Alma-Ata round table debate, during the Technical Discussions on Leadership Development for Health for All, and in informal settings. The result was the adoption of a strongly supportive resolution on Strengthening Primary Health Care, the Assembly's formal policy decision on this subject.[1] That resolution calls for further consideration by the Executive Board of WHO, and for action within WHO programmes.

These are very positive developments. The World Health Assembly, the supreme authority of WHO, has duly considered the important issues and taken definitive policy steps to ensure continued pursuit of the themes associated with the principles and intent of Alma-Ata.

That being said, can we rest assured that all has been done that can be done? Of course not! WHO itself is a large and complex organization that is very progressive in self-assessment, and recognizes the need to question its own efficiency and effectiveness. Beyond WHO, most of the actions required to advance the cause of equity are to be taken by others — nations, agencies, individuals — and resolutions passed in Geneva do not mean automatic compliance elsewhere.

A key observation at Riga was that problems that have been resistant to solution in the past, and new problems of the present, as well as others that will emerge in the future, may not be susceptible to approaches that have been applied in the past. New approaches are needed — new analyses, new mechanisms, new partnerships, new resources.

Thus, while the debates and resolutions of WHO are essential steps, they are not enough. By themselves, they will not generate sufficient creativity, resources, political strength and social energy to move through the complex thickets of severe underdevelopment, political resistance, professional disdain and social apathy. WHO can initiate, emphasize, urge and stimulate action, but, in the end, implementation must take place at community and country level.

At Riga and throughout the Assembly, there was a strong sense of progress and accomplishment with respect to health for all and equity. But there were also voices of concern that such progress and accomplishment had taken place in many but certainly not all countries.

It is important, therefore, to be very careful in assessing the prospects for health for all, and in discerning the further steps that are required. Indeed,

---

[1] See Annex 1.

in order to appreciate the full weight of the challenge before us, it is necessary to ask whether the entire effort associated with health for all may not be at risk; whether the momentum that has been built up over the past decade may not continue; whether the cynicism, materialism, militarism and plain disinterest in the problems of underdevelopment may not simply erode the spirit and energy underlying health for all.

In examining the prospects for health for all, let us be neither falsely optimistic nor morbidly pessimistic. Rather, let us look for problems and opportunities that call us to action, to sustain the strengths, to correct the weaknesses. A particular responsibility rests with us who understand the importance of the health for all movement — to be alert to those strengths and weaknesses, and to take action accordingly.

Returning to the actions recommended at Riga, which were strongly supported in discussions and by resolution in the World Health Assembly, key points can be identified, and critical questions asked that may help to focus on what lies ahead. Each area specified at Riga contains actions that are essential for health for all. Yet, looking ahead, each has uncertain strengths and an inherent unpredictability.

This will not be a detailed analysis of the actions recommended at Riga, but rather a probing at the implications of those actions, a searching for patterns of oversight and response that are called for. In the sections that follow, for each action from Riga, the opening statement is repeated (in bold type), followed by reflections that emerged at the Assembly on the implications for the future of those actions.

Actions recommended at Riga: focal points for future concern and action

---

I. Maintaining health for all as a permanent goal of all nations up to and beyond the year 2000

Reaffirm health for all as the permanent goal of all nations, as stressed in the Declaration of Alma-Ata, and establish a process for examining the longer-term challenges to health for all that will extend into the twenty-first century.

In every nation there will be continuously changing patterns of health and disease, and always there is the national responsibility for dealing with those problems in a way that safeguards the health of the people, ensures equity, and promotes a spirit of self-reliance.

It is necessary to look over the horizon, beyond the turn of the century to the problems of that time, some continuing from the present, others emerging as entirely new. The capacity for dealing with those problems needs to be strengthened further between now and the year 2000. It is likely that a very important long-term contribution of the health for all movement will be to establish in every country, and in every community, an evolving capacity to deal with the health problems of that place and time.

A critical question is: will the spirit of health for all and the quest for equity become so deeply rooted in national purposes and development processes that they will persist, that they will be sustained over time in the face of counter-forces that move against equity and ignore the poor? Will the values inherent in health for all become a permanent part of national resolve, so that they are even stronger in the next century than in this? It will be necessary to develop signals to indicate that this may be failing to take place, that those values are losing their roots and risk being blown away by the dry winds of cynicism and materialism.

II. Renewing and strengthening strategies for health for all

Encourage each country to continue to monitor its own health problems and develop its own health strategies in the spirit of health for all. This will reveal its most pressing health problems and identify the most seriously underserved and vulnerable populations. Programmes should be directed towards those populations in a spirit of equity, inviting their active participation in the development and implementation of the strategies.

The concept of health for all has provided the countries of the world with moral, political, social and technical guidelines that have enabled and encouraged them to deal more effectively with the problems of health inequity of their populations, and to serve as a basis for national strategies for health for all.

An important component of such strategies would be to establish and pursue targets for reducing disparities in both health status and access to health services between disadvantaged population groups and the general population, for example, by reducing the differences from the national mean in under-five mortality rates, infant mortality rates and maternal mortality rates.

Other forms of monitoring might be undertaken, but serious questions have to be asked about the interest in and capacity for monitoring. The first question relates to political and administrative interest in monitoring for equity since, obviously, the finding may be that certain groups are indeed underserved, with the resultant unavoidable political choice of taking action or ignoring the finding. The second question concerns the technical capacity for such monitoring, since it will require primary health care infrastructures and data systems that are seldom in place in Third World countries. Here is the paradox — where the need is greatest, the capacity for monitoring the need is weakest. Will countries give priority to building systems that can both contribute to improved PHC and support monitoring procedures?

The start WHO has made with countries reporting on progress towards health for all is very encouraging, since it has shown that, generally speaking, countries are willing to report candidly on the indicators relating to health for all. Of course, the disadvantages of reporting national rates that obscure subnational differences are well known. The shortfalls tend to be more in the limitations of available data than in readiness to report. Here is an approach to global monitoring that can be critical to ensuring continued progress towards health for all and for detecting diversions from that trend.

III. Intensifying social and political action for health for all

Intensify the social and political action necessary to support the shifts in policy and the allocation of resources required to progress towards health for all, including the involvement of other sectors, nongovernmental organizations, communities and other interested groups to seek mechanisms for promoting new partnerships for health among them and with governments.

Political will is the key to implementing the commitments to health for all. Some countries clearly have that commitment, including the necessary budgetary and administrative implementation. Others appear to pay lip-service to the ideas without serious efforts to bring them to reality. Further, many believe there is a widespread international cynicism about underdevelopment and a lack of concern about inequities and social injustices. What is the trend? Are the principles of health for all and primary health care at risk of being obliterated by these counter-values?

There is a place for continued concern about the very nature of the development process, and for watchfulness over national and international policies that are severely disadvantageous to the poor and the vulnerable. For example, is the nature of socioeconomic development such that the proportion of those in poverty remains fixed or increases even as economic progress takes place?

There is an urgent need to challenge current international development philosophies that discount investment in health and other social sectors in favour of economic improvement only. Efforts should be undertaken to enhance the national and international climate for development support, including policies that focus on social equity rather than economic considerations alone, that recognize the long-term nature of social development, and that promote wider understanding and acceptance of the development process, including respect for the people who are involved in its implementation.

Health for all calls for a broad coalition of interests with capacities in several sectors to support health-related activities. Given the limitations of governments in coping with health needs, particularly in Third World countries, the role of nongovernmental organizations (NGOs) becomes especially important. The NGOs are a special and indispensable resource for health in the world. Their uniqueness, creativity and willingness to work in remote and difficult locations give them special qualities. Their capacity either to rise from or reach to grassroots communities makes them essential partners in community-related efforts of health development.

But NGOs also present problems. Their individuality, representation of narrow constituencies, and intense focus on particular problem areas, which are sources of their strength, make it difficult for them to organize themselves for concerted action.

Is this combination — of uniqueness that gives them strength, and independence that inhibits coordinated action — inherent in the concept of NGOs? Without doubt there is a place for efforts among the NGOs to achieve greater coherence of action in the interests of HFA.

IV. Developing and mobilizing leadership for health for all

Give strong emphasis in every country to developing and stimulating the interest and support of current and potential leaders in the health and other sectors, at community, district and national levels, in order to bring creativity, advocacy, commitment and resources to bear on the challenge of health development.

WHO has led the way in bringing together leaders from many parts of the world, encouraging them to take leadership roles and providing them with opportunities to share their leadership experience with others. This effort culminated in the Technical Discussions on Leadership Development for Health for All at the World Health Assembly.

There was consensus at the Technical Discussions that we are facing a vacuum of leadership — leadership which generates a social conscience concerned with the prevailing social injustices. It may be that too much was taken for granted at Alma-Ata when it was assumed that the Declaration and the principles of primary health care would generate moral leadership. The fundamental principles of the Declaration have not been either fully understood or internalized, and there is a sizeable gap between our commitment at Alma-Ata and what is being done in each country.

It has also become evident that managerial and technocratic approaches alone will not get us to our goals. Primary health care, above all, must become a social movement — a movement in which people in all walks of life are involved as active partners and not just as passive recipients of the so-called benefits.

Such social movements demand leadership at all levels, sharing the vision of health for all and reflecting certain essential qualities: having a social conscience that generates a genuine concern for social injustices; a collective leadership that encompasses all levels of society; an "enabling" type of leadership which believes in the inherent strength and ability of the people, thereby building self-reliance; a sharing leadership in which there is no monopolizing of power.

A critical question remains: will the momentum towards developing leadership for health for all persist in the years ahead, so that leadership builds further leadership, or will the momentum fall away, the commitment wilt and the resolve to pursue health for all dissolve? Without leaders, health for all will slip from sight. Without the spirit of health for all, the principle of equity will be lost.

Given both the hopes for persistent leadership and the questions about the strength of that persistence, it will be important to follow trends in the strength of leadership for health for all. This will require the development of a fresh set of indicators that will facilitate monitoring of those trends.

V. Empowering people

Empower people by providing information, technical support and decision-making possibilities, so as to enable them to share in opportunities and reponsibilities for action in the interest of their own health. Give special attention to the role of women in health and development.

Community empowerment has had difficulty winning a place in the international taxonomy of words and ideas. Slowly, there has emerged a widespread insistence that health must be people-centred, and that caution must be exercised in promoting health services and programmes that are imposed on people from outside or from above.

Despite the recognition of this principle, it is proving difficult to build into health programmes genuine examples of community participation in programme planning, implementation, management and evaluation. That being said, there are also enough models or prototypes of such full participation to serve as encouraging examples from which others might learn.

It is probably true that the reason community empowerment is finding a place in development processes is simply because a sense of "rightness" of the concept has spread among those involved in international development. This sense of rightness is close to the social morality underlying the spirit of health for all.

Will this sense of rightness of the idea of community empowerment persist? Are its roots so deeply engaged in the soil of development processes that they cannot be torn out? Or is it so fragile a social idea that it can be uprooted and shunted aside by contrary forces in national and international development?

There is a place here for watchfulness and protectiveness in ensuring that this concept, so critical to the evolution of human dignity, is sustained, even in the midst of poverty and vulnerability.

VI. Making intersectoral collaboration a force for health for all

Support the creation of sustained intersectoral collaboration for health by incorporating health objectives into the public policies of other sectors and activating potential mechanisms at all levels.

It is widely recognized that health is not the concern of the health sector alone, but is dependent on the actions of many social and economic sectors, both governmental and nongovernmental. Nevertheless, few innovative examples exist of sustained intersectoral collaboration for health.

Sectoral priorities and rigid administrative structures usually preclude sharing of ideas, joint planning and collaborative action. This problem has been exacerbated by weak advocacy and lack of commitment to the ideas of intersectoral collaboration by the health sector itself.

The community-based emphasis of primary health care necessarily promotes intersectoral action, as community priorities almost always cut across sectors, as with the call for education, income supplementation, improvements in sanitation, and so forth. The key here, of course, is for health care to be community-based.

Nongovernmental organizations have a flexibility for organization and action that can facilitate intersectoral programming. Here, the high walls that separate sectors in governmental bureaucracies are not often present, though NGOs do have their own sectoral interests.

A useful direction for future health development is to delineate effective prototypes for intersectoral action and then promote and monitor their wider and more equitable implementation.

Monitoring of intersectoral action for health is difficult because indicators of joint action are often lacking. Measures of changes in health status do not necessarily incorporate the actions taken to achieve those changes. Input and process measures would be more likely to reveal effectiveness of intersectoral action, such as investments to combat women's illiteracy, to establish day care for children of working mothers, improvements in environmental sanitation, etc. What is problematic here is not so much the technical problems of developing a capacity for monitoring; rather, it is the concerted interest and attention to intersectoral action for health as a priority concern.

VII. Strengthening district health systems based on primary health care

Strengthen district health systems based on primary health care, as a key action point for focusing national policies and resources and local concerns on the most pressing health needs and on underserved people.

The centre of the HFA movement is the development of health services based on PHC that can reach entire populations with services according to need, including full community participation. Since Riga, WHO has resolved to give increased emphasis to research and development in PHC with emphasis on district health systems.

What will happen between now and the turn of the century? What is the likelihood that PHC will even remotely approach universal coverage with services that are effective, affordable and culturally acceptable? Those who work in Africa and Southern Asia see the road towards universal coverage as being very long and very rocky. Political commitment to these issues is now virtually universal, but full budgetary support, administrative perseverance, and expert knowledge about how to bring PHC to operational effectiveness are much less consistent.

None the less, there are examples where PHC has taken hold with substantial impact on health indicators. Thailand provides an example, where the effort has gone beyond health for all to widespread community involvement in pursuing quality of life through a multisectoral approach.

In Nigeria, there have been substantial shifts in national health policy towards community-based PHC, and the country appears to be swinging towards increased effectiveness of PHC. Further, Nigeria has attracted support from progressive donors who are interested in supporting comprehensive approaches to PHC development, including PHC infrastructure development.

The district focus for research and development, newly emphasized by WHO, grounded as it is in the workings of government and close to the people, brings a new practicality to this field of work.

It would seem, therefore, that there is an international need for monitoring progress toward more effective PHC systems, including particularly the development of prototypes or models and the dissemination of these concepts and prototypes, and for encouraging donors to support more comprehensive approaches to PHC, including infrastructure development and strong community involvement.

VIII. Planning, preparing and supporting health personnel for health for all

Reorient education and training programmes for health personnel, emphasizing relevance to health services requirements, by locating learning experiences in functioning health systems based on primary health care. Provide strong moral and resource support for personnel, particularly those working in remote areas or difficult circumstances.

From among the many issues that could be discussed about human resource development, two can be used to illustrate both the potential and the problems of this field of concern: the relevance of preparation of manpower to health services needs, and the role of universities in that interaction.

The critical relationships in human resource development involve the interaction of manpower development and health services requirements. Planning, preparation and utilization must be closely integrated. While there is general understanding of these principles, such logical interaction is not the usual mode, either because those who plan for and use manpower are not closely related to those who prepare them, or because there is a lack of interest in the interaction. The sad story is that in much of the world, doctors are not prepared for, interested in or competent to deal with the broader health problems of the populations their educational programmes are intended to serve.

The International Conference on Health Manpower Out of Balance, sponsored by CIOMS and WHO in Acapulco, Mexico, September 1986, apparently had a striking impact on countries that had given little attention to linkages between preparation of and needs for health manpower, and particularly those that had allowed a health manpower glut to develop.

The full responsibility for such irrelevance does not rest with universities alone, but the potential of universities to deal with the issues is very large. There is a widespread impression, however, that many, perhaps most universities, particularly medical colleges, are not closely interested in or even sensitive to these issues. Or if interest is professed, it does not result in changes in curriculum and practice that would promise much impact on health.

There are favourable indicators as well. The Network of Community-Oriented Educational Institutions for Health Sciences represents a highly innovative effort to influence health sciences institutions towards community-oriented and problem-based approaches to learning. Further, the World Conference on Medical Education held in Edinburgh in August 1988 was an important milestone in this effort. The WHO Regional Office for Europe is in the early stages of developing "health for all" curricula for both medical schools and schools of public health. Some individual institutions refer to themselves as health-for-all universities.[1]

Here, then, are mixed signals about these two critical issues: relevance of preparation of manpower to health services needs, and the roles of universities in that interaction. It will be important to follow and monitor the trends. This leaves open the question of the steps to be taken if trends are away from principles relating to equity in health.

IX. Ensuring the development and rational use of science and appropriate technology

Emphasize the applications of science and appropriate technology to the critical health problems that threaten populations in all parts of the world, and strengthen the research capacities of Third World countries, with emphasis on research aimed at improving the health of the most deprived people.

Science has much to offer the pursuit of health for all. Some problems call for advanced scientific insight and methodologies almost on an emergency scale, as in grappling with the AIDS pandemic. There are other calls on science, some less dramatic, but no less important, for example, applications of diagnostic methods that can be used in remote locations. New vaccines will strengthen health services, and new techniques for the control of tropical diseases will ease the burden of suffering on countless lives.

However, the most serious deficiencies in improving health in developing countries do not relate to shortages of technology, but to inadequacies of health system infrastructures and the high costs of making technology available to all in need. This fundamental deficiency is often compounded by the indiscriminate transfer of technology to developing countries.

Assessment of the costs and impacts of alternative technologies has an important place. The costs of the transfer of technology may be more than that of the technology itself.

Most health problems of developing countries cannot be solved by indiscriminate technology transfer. Solutions must be developed on the spot, and capacity-building in research is essential, based on a clear view of the range of technological choices involved, and a detailed knowledge of local research capacities.

The need for a balanced strategy is clear: where there is continued alertness for advances in technology that are applicable to Third World countries,

---

[1] See page 58

recognizing that adaptations will be necessary; where there is continued effort to extend health services infrastructures to the social and geographic periphery so the benefits of science and technology can be spread equitably; and where there is increasing effort to strengthen research capacities of Third World countries.

Such balance provides guidance for monitoring the rational uses of science and technology so as to ensure that transfers of technology are not indiscriminate and blind to local priority needs, that health services reach those in need and carry applicable technology to them, and that research-capacity building is not only emphasized in relation to Third World problems but also takes place in Third World settings.

X. Overcoming problems that continue to resist solution

Establish priority programmes aimed at overcoming serious problems, where underdevelopment or disturbances in development are major contributing factors and progress has been very limited, such as high infant, child and maternal mortality rates, abuse of substances such as tobacco and alcohol, and the imbalance between population growth and environmental and socioeconomic resources. Develop improved approaches through primary health care, emphasizing intersectoral action.

The most serious problems to be addressed between now and the year 2000 will be those that resist solution largely because of underlying conditions of severe underdevelopment, as in the least developed countries, or long-established patterns of personal and social behaviour, as in developed countries. It is necessary to be clear, however, that the people are not the causes of these problems, they are the victims, and solutions must address development problems at their roots, and not simply blame people for circumstances the world has given them.

Consideration needs to be given to the reasons why many health problems are resistant to solution. Progress has been slow in dealing with many of these problems, despite growing understanding of the problems, progress in health service development and the steady emergence of new technologies.

Obviously, the reasons for lack of progress are multifactorial — solutions are at hand but the health service infrastructure fails to reach the people; the technology is available but not understood by those who must implement it; the system is there but is so poorly managed as to be in a state of chronic failure; the political and administrative commitments are weak or absent; health-based solutions are inadequate when development itself has "gone wrong", as in severe ecological deterioration associated with excessive population growth.

A critical point in this context is that current approaches are falling short. The health machinery of today — local, national, global — is not adequate. New approaches are needed. New indicators of action and impact are required. There is a need to move on to new ground, but taking new directions is difficult, and will be done only if there is the continued conviction of the importance of addressing the problems of severe underdevelopment to reach those who have no voice to claim our attention, and our creative attack on their problems.

Special priority initiative in support of the least developed countries by WHO and the international community

> **Establish a special international initiative focused on the tragic circumstances of the least developed countries, mostly on the continent of Africa, and especially those with markedly elevated infant, under-five-year-old and maternal mortality rates, which will address specific obstacles to progress and will set targets to be reached by the year 2000.**

While most countries have benefited from the health for all movement, a tragic residue is suffering from death and disability so extreme as to leave no doubt that they are being bypassed by even the barest opportunities to progress towards a minimal level of human dignity and well-being.

Here is the hard core of the challenge in health development — extreme technological difficulties to be faced under conditions of severe underdevelopment. It was with respect to these countries that Dr Grant asked, "Shouldn't we insist that the still massive death rates of children be placed along with slavery, colonialism, racism and apartheid, on the shelf reserved for those things which are simply no longer acceptable to humankind?"

At Riga, the feeling was strong that WHO and the international community should focus special concern on the plight of the least developed countries. The further point was made that the World Health Assembly should undertake to monitor the outcomes of this effort, and that the rate of progress should serve as an indicator of the effectiveness of the resolve of the Member States in dealing with this most fundamental of challenges — the countries that, without effective development assistance and collaboration, will probably slip further down the spiral of development failure.

The Health Assembly did, indeed, express special concern for the least developed countries in its resolution on Strengthening Primary Health Care.[1] Given the depth and complexity of the problems, many of them cross-sectoral in nature, it will be necessary to focus on how that monitoring is to be done, what the indicators are to be, and who the responsible parties will be.

---

[1] See Annex 1.

While these are challenging issues, the facts that WHO has generally accepted the actions recommended at Riga and has decided to give special attention to the least developed countries, including monitoring of progress in dealing with their problems, are of extraordinary importance. It means that the issue of extreme inequities in health and development is taken seriously by WHO and its Member States. The concrete steps of responding to this call to action lie ahead.

A twofold agenda for
the year 2000 and beyond

What have the recommendations from Riga and the responses from the World Health Assembly told us about Alma-Ata and its call for health for all based on primary health care? What have they told us about social morality and the resolve of the Member States of WHO with respect to the needs of the poorest and most vulnerable of our world? They have told us that we have a chance. Nothing more. No guarantees. No assurances. We cannot know that we will in fact push back the obstacles to health for all and replace them with even a semblance of equity in health. But the possibility that we have a chance of having an impact on this portion of our world's problems is a very special insight indeed.

The opposite was possible (many would have said a certainty) — that the notion of a new form of social morality in health was too faint and fragile to take hold, and that a decade of global effort would prove the hopelessness of such dreaming. But such is not the case, as affirmed by dozens upon dozens of nations, organizations and individuals, who insisted that the gains have been widespread, substantial and repeated.

With the affirmations, however, came hard facts — of unevenness of progress in virtually all countries, of partial successes, unsolved problems, and newly emerging problems. Of central concern are those untouched by health for all and primary health care — the tragic residuum of the poorest of the poor in the least developed countries, largely abandoned to their poverty and despair.

Riga made the point emphatically that a number of problems are proving to be resistant to solution, and that WHO and its Member States must develop new approaches to them. This perspective was absorbed into the debates at the World Health Assembly and incorporated into the resolution on Strengthening Primary Health Care.

During the round table debate on the tenth anniversary of Alma-Ata, the Moderator, Sir John Reid, asked the participants: "Has Alma-Ata made a difference?" Dr Al-Awadi responded to the question by saying emphatically that it most certainly has, and then went on to say that the principles from Alma-Ata and the social morality they represent are so important to the world that they must be watched and protected, and that a Board of Trustees for Health for All is therefore necessary.

Considerable informal discussion has followed Dr Al-Awadi's suggestion, including the possibility that an international mechanism might be established to carry out the monitoring or auditing function implicit in the concept of a Board of Trustees. Alternative language was suggested — that the monitoring and protective function might be called an International Watch for Health and Equity, or, within WHO, an Advisory or Oversight Committee on Health and Equity.

145

Thus, looking ahead to the year 2000 and beyond, a twofold agenda has emerged.

Responding to the challenge — building health systems based on primary health care

Riga built the case for fresh approaches to an inventory of difficult problems, some that have proven resistant to solution, others newly emerging. The World Health Assembly resolution on Strengthening Primary Health Care provides a renewed policy basis for moving ahead and marshalling the resources of WHO and the entire international community to deal with these residual and evolving problems.

Here is the immense challenge to build on the experience of the past decade and before, and to ensure that the most creative of our energies go into the continued improvement of health systems based on the primary health care approach. This challenge is directed towards the needs of all people, but with particular concern for those who are most vulnerable and most in need, as exemplified by the poorest people in the least developed countries where mortality rates are up to 100 times those of the developed world.

There is no reason to doubt that this can be done, given the chance to address the problems in an international atmosphere of conviction that this is a global priority. The creativity is there. The resilience is there. What is needed is the chance.

Protecting the chance — ensuring that priority is given to equity in health

How can we be sure of the chance, that the international resolve to deal with these problems on a priority basis will persist, that the concept of social morality and concern for the poor, neglected and helpless will be strengthened and not diminished?

Dr Al-Awadi's call for a Board of Trustees implies a monitoring or oversight function that will somehow reflect the conviction of the community of nations that this priority for the poorest people in the poorest nations is inherently right, and that there is no acceptable alternative strategy.

Dr Mahler said at the Health Assembly, "We must have a moral obsession about the least developed countries. They are missing out totally on the development process. It is development-gone-wrong. They must be brought on board in a real and true sense before the year 2000. But not just to survive in misery, but survival in which their children can realize their physical, social and spiritual potential."

The Board of Trustees would provide a further means of responding to Dr Mahler's call for a moral obsession in relation to the least developed countries, and to Mr Grant's for rejecting massive deaths of children as simply unacceptable to humankind.

Two approaches can be envisioned. One would be to establish a formal mechanism, such as an international body — a commission, perhaps — recognized by international agencies, NGOs and governments, and functioning in close cooperation with them, possibly within WHO itself. The other would be to formulate an international code of principles and values that would constitute guidelines for the content of international and national policies and programmes to ensure continued pursuit of equity in health.

Perhaps the most salient question at this point would be: Is a Board of Trustees really necessary? This question is reminiscent of other discussions of requirements for a viable future for the world in which the conviction has been expressed that, barring nuclear catastrophe, the real risks to the possibility of mankind proceeding safely into the future are not ecological disasters or failure to feed growing populations; they are technical problems susceptible to solution. The most serious risks lie in the failure to develop effective international mechanisms for governing the interactions of people and nations on a global scale in an era in which there is growing complexity of interaction, increasing rapidity of change, and dangerously shortened decision times.

Analogously, we can say that the technical aspects of even the most intractable health problems that face us can be overcome. The international community of nations has the ingenuity and resources for doing so. Even the rapidity of progress in dealing with such difficult problems as immunizing the world's children has been startling — one example of the global capacity to address critical problems. AIDS comes to mind immediately as an extraordinary threat to health in our comtemporary world, but hardly anyone expects us to fail in ultimately controlling the problem.

No, the critical ingredients for equity in health in the long term are not technical; rather, they have to do with international resolve, with fundamental belief and conviction in what are the right things to do. But it is also likely that resolve and conviction by themselves would be relatively ineffective in guiding and controlling major divergences from internationally accepted principles. It would be naive to believe otherwise.

The case can be made, therefore, looking to the year 2000 and beyond, that the most serious risks for failure in achieving some semblance of equity in health lie not in the failure to respond technologically to the difficult problems of implementing the primary health care approach, but rather in the failure to develop effective international mechanisms for guiding or governing the implementation of principles to which the global community of nations has agreed, and for maintaining that commitment as a code of values that is diffused throughout development policies and programmes.

A new form of international dialogue?

Mechanisms might be proposed for safeguarding the principles of health for all and equity in health. But by the very nature of those mechanisms, the basis for such protection is moral suasion. In the end, the forces involved are neither stronger nor weaker than the international conviction of the rightness of the issue.

How strong might these forces be, or might they become?

Attempts to use moral suasion around such issues is not new in the world, and the record of its effectiveness is mixed, but not without examples of substantial impact.

Further, some recent events call attention to the possibility that there may be opportunities for new kinds of dialogue in the development field:

- The debates and actions around economic adjustment in connection with financial assistance to developing countries, which was initially implemented more or less blind to the impact on vulnerable populations, but with a later tilt toward protection of those groups, generated by international criticism and discussion.

- The slow shift of health services development strategy towards: (1) *community* self-reliance in planning and decision-making, which represents some degree of yielding of control by health professionals; and (2) *national* self-reliance in planning and decision-making, which represents some yielding of control by donor agencies.

- The implementation of essential drugs policies, which have proceeded from bruising interactions between involved parties towards positions likely to be more mutually beneficial.

With respect to equity, and unlike some of the more conflictual interactions in the North-South arena, there are no antagonists or protagonists. It is likely that there will be universal agreement on what is desirable. The infractions and diversions will often appear more as unintended consequences of decisions to pursue other tracks of development: high-technology medical care v. primary health care, economically-oriented v. socially-oriented development, etc. Of course, there will be times when the infraction has malicious intent only thinly disguised as a competing form of development, e.g. the marketing of tobacco products.

The point is that here is a possibility that all parties committed to equity in health — international organizations, governments, NGOs, industry — will gather around this issue, formulate broadly acceptable principles, and welcome a mechanism for monitoring their application, as well as promoting constructive responses to infractions or shortfalls.

References

1. Tagore, R. *Glimpses of Bengal: Selected letters, 1885-1895.* New Delhi, Macmillan, 1980, pp. 102-103.
2. World Health Organization. *Handbook of resolutions and decisions,* Vol. II, 1973-1984. Geneva, 1985, p. 1.
3. World Health Organization. *Evaluation of the strategy for health for all by the year 2000: Seventh report on the world health situation.* Geneva, 1987.
4. UNICEF. *The state of the world's children, 1987.* New York, Oxford University Press, 1987.
5. UNICEF. *The state of the world's children, 1988.* New York, Oxford University Press, 1988.
6. World Bank. *World development report, 1987.* London, Oxford University Press, 1987.
7. Reid, Sir John. Alma-Ata and after — the background. In: *Primary health care 2000.* Edinburgh, Churchill Livingstone, 1986, pp. 3-16.
8. World Health Organization. *Alma-Ata 1978: Primary health care.* Geneva, 1978 ("Health for All" Series, No. 1).
9. World Health Organization. *Global strategy for health for all by the year 2000.* Geneva, 1981 ("Health for All" Series, No. 3).
10. UNICEF. *The state of the world's children, 1987.* New York, Oxford University Press, 1987, p. 45.
11. World Health Organization. *Evaluation of the strategy for health for all by the year 2000: Seventh report on the world health situation. Vol. 1: Global review.* Geneva, 1987, p. 113.
12. UNICEF. *The state of the world's children, 1988.* New York, Oxford University Press, 1988, pp. 64-65.
13. UNICEF. *The state of the world's children, 1987.* New York, Oxford University Press, 1987, p. 7.
14. *Targets for health for all: Targets in support of the European strategy for health for all.* Copenhagen, WHO Regional Office for Europe, 1985.
15. World Health Organization. *Evaluation of the strategy for health for all by the year 2000: Seventh report on the world health situation. Vol. 5: European Region.* Copenhagen, 1986, pp. v-vi.
16. Lalonde, M. *A new perspective on the health of Canadians: a working document.* Ottawa, Department of National Health and Welfare, 1977.
17. World Health Organization. *Evaluation of the strategy for health for all by the year 2000: Seventh report on the world health situation. Vol. 3: Region of the Americas.* Washington, DC, 1986, pp. 86-90.
18. United States Public Health Service, Office of Health Promotion and Disease Prevention. *Health objectives for the nation.* Washington, DC, 1986.
19. Sidel, V. W. The fabric of public health: 1985 presidential address, annual meeting of the American Public Health Association, Washington, DC. *American journal of public health,* 76(4): 373-378 (1986).

20. World Health Organization. *Evaluation of the strategy for health for all by the year 2000: Seventh report on the world health situation. Vol. 1: Global review.* Geneva, 1987, pp. 81-82.

21. World Health Organization. *Evaluation of the strategy for health for all by the year 2000: Seventh report on the world health situation. Vol. 5: European Region.* Copenhagen, 1986, p. 4.

22. McKeown, T. *The role of medicine: dream, mirage or nemesis?* Oxford, Blackwell, 1979.

23. Chanawongse, K. & Singhadej, O. From primary health care to basic minimum needs and quality of life; the challenge for MIS in Thailand. In: *Management information systems and microcomputers in primary health care:* Report of an International Workshop, Lisbon, November 1987. Geneva, Aga Khan Foundation, 1988.

24. Brown, L. R. & Wolf, E. C. Charting a sustainable course. In: *State of the world 1987: Worldwatch Institute report on progress toward a sustainable society.* New York, Norton, 1987, p. 203.

25. Caldwell, J. C. Routes to low mortality in poor countries. *Population and development review,* **12**(2): 171-220 (1986).

26. Brown, L. R. & Jacobson, J. L. *The future of urbanization: Facing the ecological and economic constraints.* Washington, DC, Worldwatch Institute, 1987 (Worldwatch Paper 77).

27. UNICEF. *The state of the world's children, 1988.* New York, Oxford University Press, 1988, pp. 64-65 and 76-77.

28. Briend, A. et al. Usefulness of nutritional indices and classification in predicting deaths of malnourished children. *British medical journal,* **293**: 373-375 (1986).

29. Chen, L. C. Malnutrition and mortality. *Bulletin of the Nutrition Foundation of India,* October 1982.

30. Brown, L. R. Analyzing the demographic trap. In: *State of the world 1987: Worldwatch Institute report on progress toward a sustainable society.* New York, Norton, 1987, pp. 20-37.

31. World Health Organization. *Evaluation of the strategy for health for all by the year 2000: Seventh report on the world health situation. Vol. 4: South-East Asia Region.* New Delhi, 1987, pp. 8-9.

32. World Health Organization. *Evaluation of the strategy for health for all by the year 2000: Seventh report on the world health situation. Vol. 3: Region of the Americas.* Washington, DC, 1986, pp. 15 and 155.

33. World Health Organization. *Evaluation of the strategy for health for all by the year 2000: Seventh report on the world health situation. Vol. 5: European Region.* Copenhagen, 1986, pp. 110, 118, 192 and 296.

34. Bankowski, Z. & Bryant, J. H., ed. *Health policy, ethics and human values: An international dialogue.* Geneva, CIOMS, 1985.

35. UNICEF. *The state of the world's children, 1987.* New York, Oxford University Press, 1987, pp. 2 and 4.

36. UNICEF. *The state of the world's children, 1988.* New York, Oxford University Press, 1988, pp. 74-75.

37. Pew Memorial Trust/World Bank/WHO. *International health policy research program.* Washington, DC, 1987.

38. Josephs, D. & Middleton, J. D. Arms or health? *Lancet,* 28 November 1987.

39. Smith, D. L. & Bryant, J. H. Building the infrastructure for primary health care: An overview of vertical and integrated approaches. *Social science and medicine,* **26:**909-917 (1988).

40. Rifkin, S. & Walt, G. Editorial: The debate on selective or comprehensive primary health care. *Social science and medicine,* **26:**877-878 (1988).

41. WHO Technical Report Series, No. 744, 1987 (*Hospitals and health for all:* report of a WHO Expert Committee).

42. Reynolds, J. et al. Community PHC management information systems: guidelines for development of a model system. In: *Management information systems and microcomputers in primary health care:* Report of an International Workshop, Lisbon, November 1987. Geneva, Aga Khan Foundation, 1988.

43. UNICEF. *The state of the world's children, 1988.* New York, Oxford University Press, 1988, pp. 31-37.

44. Bankowski, Z. & Bryant, J. H., ed. *Health policy, ethics and human values: European and North American perspectives.* Geneva, CIOMS, 1988.

45. WHO Technical Report Series, No. 717, 1985 (*Health manpower requirements for the achievement of health for all by the year 2000 through primary health care:* report of a WHO Expert Committee).

46. Bankowski, Z. & Mejia, A., ed. *Health manpower out of balance: Conflicts and prospects.* Geneva, CIOMS, 1987.

47. WHO Technical Report Series, No. 708, 1984 (*Education and training of nurse teachers and managers with special regard to primary health care:* report of a WHO Expert Committee), p. 84.

48. Bryant, J. H. Health services, health manpower, and universities in relation to health for all: An historical and future perspective. *American journal of public health,* **74**: 714-719 (1984).

Annex 1

Resolution WHA41.34:
Strengthening primary health care

The Forty-first World Health Assembly,

Recalling resolution WHA30.43 in which it was decided that the main social target of governments and WHO should be the attainment by all the people of the world by the year 2000 of a level of health that will permit them to lead a socially and economically productive life;

Further recalling resolution WHA32.30 which endorsed the Declaration of Alma-Ata with its emphasis on primary health care and its integrated approach as the key to attaining health for all, and resolution WHA34.36 by which the Health Assembly adopted the Global Strategy for Health for All by the Year 2000;

Mindful of United Nations General Assembly resolution 36/43 which endorsed the Global Strategy, urged all Member States to ensure its implementation as part of their multisectoral development efforts, and requested all appropriate organizations and bodies of the United Nations system to collaborate with WHO in carrying it out;

Having considered the statement issued by a meeting in Riga, Union of Soviet Socialist Republics, in March 1988 to mark the tenth anniversary of the Declaration of Alma-Ata, known as "Alma-Ata reaffirmed at Riga";

Recognizing that, at this mid-point between the establishment and the attainment of the goal of health for all by the year 2000, much progress has been made by many countries in parallel with the evolution of their social and economic situation, but that there remain a considerable number of countries in which the health situation and the means for improving it remain highly unsatisfactory ten years after Alma-Ata;

Convinced of the importance of district health systems for the optimal organization and provision of primary health care, as an integral part of national health systems and of the global health system and constructed primarily by countries themselves with appropriate support by WHO, as well as of the need for research and development as a vital step in fostering the development of such care;

Recognizing further that the active participation of the people and the communities and their contribution are essential to the attainment of the goal of health for all;

1. ENDORSES the statement "Alma-Ata reaffirmed at Riga", which emphasizes that the Declaration of Alma-Ata remains valid for all countries at all stages of social and economic development and that the application of its principles should therefore be maintained after the year 2000;

2. URGES all Member States:

   (1) to increase their efforts to attain the goal of health for all by the year 2000 through health systems based on primary health care in line with the

global, regional and national strategies to that end, taking into account the statement "Alma-Ata reaffirmed at Riga";

(2) to prepare for the continuation of these efforts beyond the year 2000 to ensure the maintenance and progressive improvement of the health of all their people;

3. THANKS all the multilateral and bilateral development agencies, nongovernmental organizations and voluntary and philanthropic bodies that have supported the struggle to attain health for all and appeals to them to continue and intensify this support;

4. CALLS ON the international community:

(1) to continue its support to the efforts of Member States in the development of health systems based on primary health care;

(2) to take unprecedented measures to support the least developed countries committed to improving the health of their people in line with the policy of health for all;

(3) to support such efforts under the international coordination of WHO;

5. REQUESTS the regional committees:

(1) to pay particular attention to the monitoring and evaluation of strategies for health for all, with a view to identifying areas in which particular efforts are required and to taking appropriate action;

(2) to report thereon to the Executive Board in conformity with the revised plan of action for implementing the Global Strategy for Health for All;

6. REQUESTS the Director-General:

(1) to ensure the widest dissemination of this resolution and the statement "Alma-Ata reaffirmed at Riga";

(2) to cooperate with Member States in the implementation of the recommendations made at Riga for accelerating progress towards health for all by the year 2000, paying particular attention to the problems that have hitherto resisted solution;

(3) to intensify the programme of activities of research and development in primary health care, including health services, within the existing organizational framework, with particular emphasis on:

(a) strengthening integrated health approaches and district health systems within the national context;

(b) the development and rational use of science and appropriate technology and their transfer among countries;

(4) to secure resources from within the regular budget of the Organization and the continued mobilization of extrabudgetary resources as additional means for implementation of the above programme;

(5) to ensure that the activities of the programme and those of all other related programmes give particular emphasis to supporting the least developed countries;

153

(6) to direct all programmes of the Organization to increase their support to countries in strengthening the integrated approach and in research and development in primary health care, with emphasis on strengthening district health systems;

(7) to present to the Executive Board at its eighty-third session proposals for intensification of activities of research and development in primary health care, including the feasibility of establishing a special programme, and information on international support to the least developed countries;

7. REQUESTS the Executive Board:

(1) to intensify its monitoring and evaluation of the Global Strategy for Health for All, paying particular attention to supporting countries in the strengthening of integrated approaches and to international support to the least developed countries;

(2) to report on this subject to the Health Assembly in conformity with the revised plan of action for implementing the Global Strategy for Health for All.

Annex 2

Resolution WHA41.26:
Leadership development for health for all

The Forty-first World Health Assembly,

Recalling resolutions WHA30.43 and WHA34.36 by which the Member States of WHO unanimously adopted a policy and strategy for achieving the goal of health for all by the year 2000;

Noting the progress made at this midpoint between the adoption in 1978 of the Declaration of Alma-Ata on Primary Health Care, which set a new course for action for health, and the year 2000, but also being aware of the need for accelerated progress to achieve the collectively agreed goal of health for all;

Stressing that accelerated progress will require an even greater involvement of people from all walks of life and the mobilization of all potential resources in society in support of primary health care;

Recognizing that informed and committed leadership at all levels of society is crucial for harnessing this potential;

Recalling resolution WHA37.31 on the role of universities in the strategies for health for all, resolution WHA38.31 on collaboration with nongovernmental organizations in implementing the strategy, resolution WHA39.7 on the evaluation of the strategy, and resolution WHA39.22 on intersectoral action for health;

1. ENDORSES the Declaration of Personal Commitment[1] and the report of the Technical Discussions held during the Forty-first World Health Assembly, on leadership development for health for all;

2. AFFIRMS that enlightened and effective leadership is vital to intensify and sustain social and political action for health for all;

3. CALLS ON Member States:

   (1) to develop leadership for health for all actively by using all educational entry points, and by sensitizing current leadership to the issues involved and generating continually new leadership, in order to accelerate progress towards health for all through primary health care;

   (2) to make renewed efforts to increase understanding of health for all and primary health care, utilizing effective communication strategies, including sensitizing the leadership of the media to their social responsibility in promoting communication for health;

   (3) to accelerate decentralization and socioeconomic and structural reforms which favour active involvement of people and encourage the emergence of leadership potential and provide opportunities for setting examples of effective leadership at all levels;

---

[1] Text annexed to this resolution.

(4) to make renewed and innovative efforts to involve people and communities creatively so as to empower them, develop self-reliance and leadership at local level;

(5) to expand mutually supportive partnerships with communities, nongovernmental organizations, educational institutions and other community-based organizations to bring their creativity and commitment to bear on the challenge of health for all;

4. CALLS ON the leadership of educational institutions and universities to demonstrate their commitment to achieve health for all through primary health care, by:

(1) accelerating changes in the curricula for the training of health and other professionals, including teachers, involved in health action to promote the value system of health for all and enhance the potential of leadership for health for all;

(2) shifting academic reward systems and providing career opportunities so as to acknowledge and encourage career academic commitments to primary health care;

(3) including in the curricula of institutions throughout the educational system, from primary schools on, subjects related to education for health, social values, attitudinal change and leadership development;

5. URGES the leadership of national and international nongovernmental organizations to expand their partnership with governments and educational institutions to accelerate progress towards health for all, and to use their flexibility and creativity in developing leadership potential and capacities at community level, involving particularly women and youth groups;

6. REQUESTS the Director-General:

(1) to publish the Declaration of Personal Commitment and the report of the Technical Discussions on leadership development for health for all, and disseminate them widely to all governments, educational institutions and universities, nongovernmental and voluntary organizations, and other interested groups;

(2) to ensure the continuity and sustainability of the leadership development initiative within WHO, building upon the strong beginnings already realized, and establishing other appropriate mechanisms so that it becomes an integral part of WHO's support for the health-for-all strategy, at all levels;

(3) to support the efforts of Member States, educational institutions and nongovernmental organizations in their endeavours to develop leadership to accelerate social and political action towards health for all through primary health care, and to encourage the use of WHO resources, particularly fellowships, for leadership development;

(4) to establish and foster a technical resource network drawn from educational institutions and health leaders, to provide support to health for all and leadership development;

(5) to promote and encourage leadership potential by documenting and disseminating information on successful and innovative initiatives in

primary health care and creating incentives such as awards and recognition for such endeavours, and to provide simplified and relevant documentation for lay people and community leadership;

(6) to evaluate the impact of the leadership development initiative in implementing the Global Strategy for Health for All in conjunction with the second evaluation of the strategy in 1991, and to report thereon to the eighty-ninth session of the Executive Board and the Forty-fifth World Health Assembly in 1992.

Annex to WHA41.26

Declaration of personal commitment

We, the participants at the Technical Discussions on leadership development for health for all (held in Geneva on 5-7 May 1988, during the Forty-first World Health Assembly), representing people from many walks of life, including governments, nongovernmental organizations, universities, educational institutions, voluntary agencies and United Nations agencies, make the following declaration:

I. *We believe that*:

• there is a need for greater concern and commitment to achieve the goal of health for all by the year 2000 through primary health care, among political, professional and community leaders;

• building self-reliance and leadership capabilities at local level is the most important ingredient for sustained development and progress in health;

• the development of leadership that can be sustained as a continuing process at all levels is an important strategy to mobilize greater social and political commitment for the total health-for-all movement.

II. *We therefore commit ourselves* and urge others in leadership and other strategic positions to adopt the following *Five-point Personal Agenda for Action*:

1. to *inform* ourselves, our colleagues, fellow-workers, community members and others about the fundamental values, principles and processes to achieve health for all by the year 2000 through primary health care, and to *generate a social conscience in people* regarding the health conditions and needs of the under-served, socially deprived and vulnerable population groups;

2. to make a serious *review* of progress towards the specific targets set in our respective countries, to identify where the critical needs and gaps are, and to *provide leadership* in identifying and implementing corrective actions;

3. to serve as *prime movers* for change, particularly in areas which fall within our respective roles, and to *motivate others* to accelerate the changes required in order to achieve the goal of health for all;

4. to develop and promote *partnerships* and new alliances of support for health, including the professional associations, institutions of higher education, religious leaders, people's organizations, concerned non-governmental organizations and individuals, philanthropic groups, the private sector and the media;

5. to promote *self-reliance* and *enable others,* particularly within the home and at the community level, to take greater responsibility for their own health and the health of their communities, through informing and educating them and developing their leadership potential.

III. *We are convinced that* additional courageous and innovative strategies and tactics will be needed to ensure that all people of the world will be covered by primary health care. Leadership development is one such strategy which provides new opportunities to inform and communicate, to expand partnerships among people — people who are empowered and motivated — who then take on new responsibilities for their health, the health of their families and of their communities.